Hawraa Mahmood Murad
Rawaa Safaa Abbas AL_Azzawi
Mariam Kazim Jassab

Pathology and Physiology in Animals: From Function to Disease..

Hawraa Mahmood Murad
Rawaa Safaa Abbas AL_Azzawi
Mariam Kazim Jassab

Pathology and Physiology in Animals: From Function to Disease..

Noor Publishing

Imprint
Any brand names and product names mentioned in this book are subject to trademark, brand or patent protection and are trademarks or registered trademarks of their respective holders. The use of brand names, product names, common names, trade names, product descriptions etc. even without a particular marking in this work is in no way to be construed to mean that such names may be regarded as unrestricted in respect of trademark and brand protection legislation and could thus be used by anyone.

Cover image: www.ingimage.com

Publisher:
Noor Publishing
is a trademark of
Dodo Books Indian Ocean Ltd. and OmniScriptum S.R.L publishing group

120 High Road, East Finchley, London, N2 9ED, United Kingdom
Str. Armeneasca 28/1, office 1, Chisinau MD-2012, Republic of Moldova, Europe
Managing Directors: Ieva Konstantinova, Victoria Ursu
info@omniscriptum.com

Printed at: see last page
ISBN: 978-620-9-56246-4

Pathology and Physiology in Animals: From Function to Disease

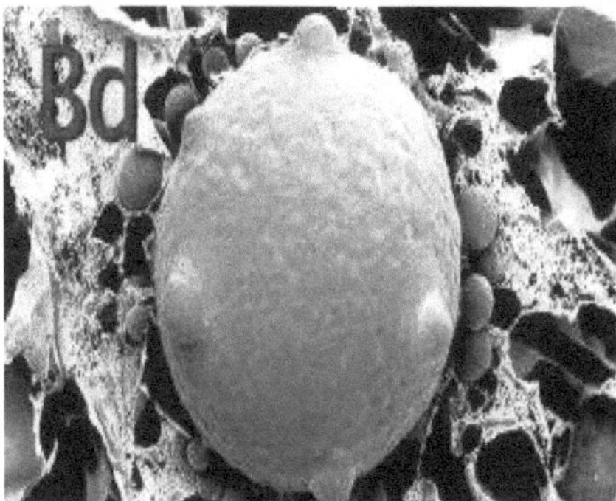

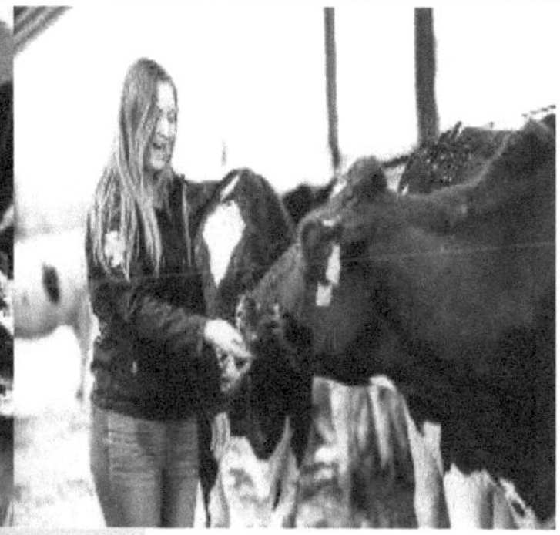

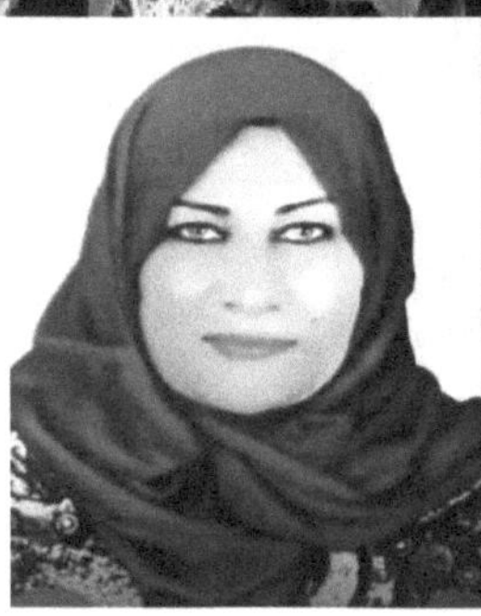

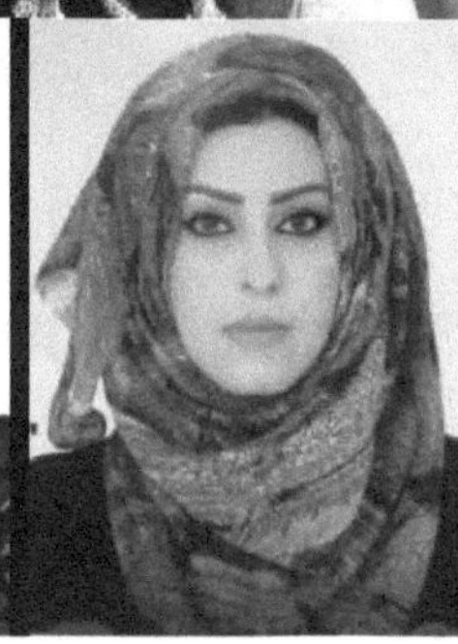

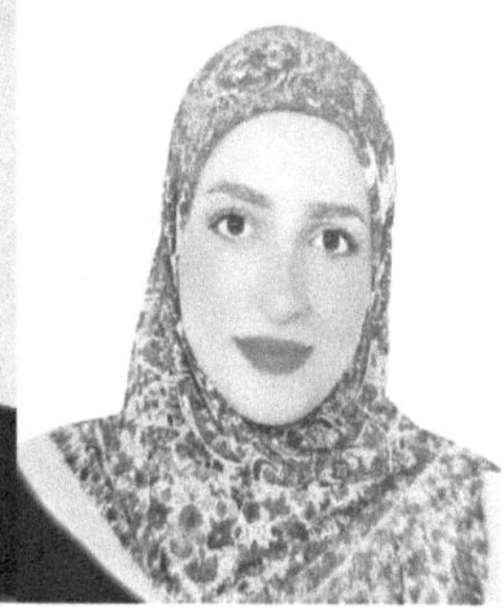

By

Dr. Hawraa Mahmood Murad

Dr. Rawaa Safaa Abbas AL_Azzawi

Dr. Mariam Kazim Jassab

(2026)

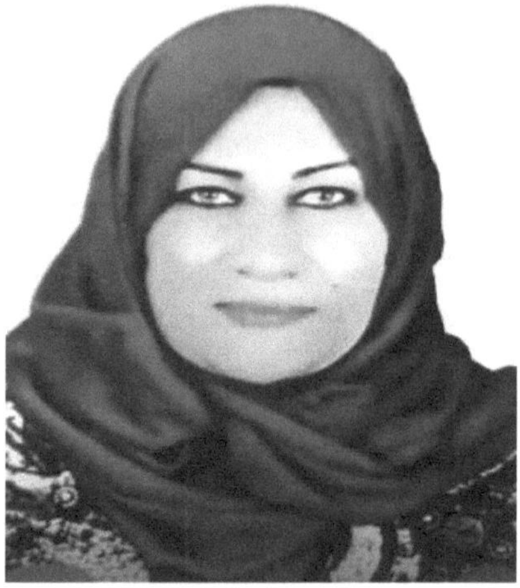

Dr. Hawraa Mahmood Murad

Department of biology, College of science, Al-Qasim Green University, Iraq

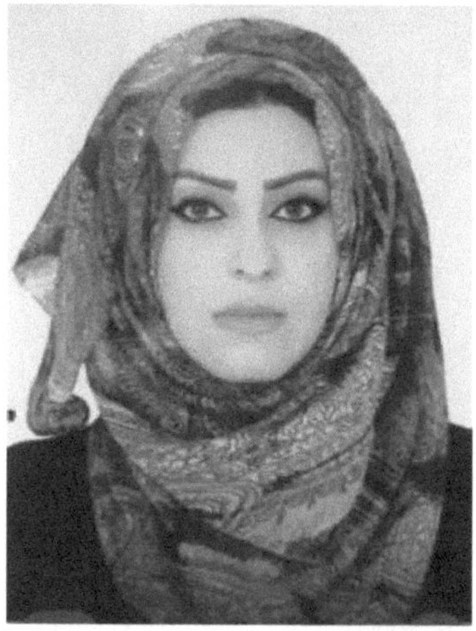

Dr. Rawaa Safaa Abbas AL_Azzawi

Department of biology, Collage of science, Al-Qasim Green University, Iraq

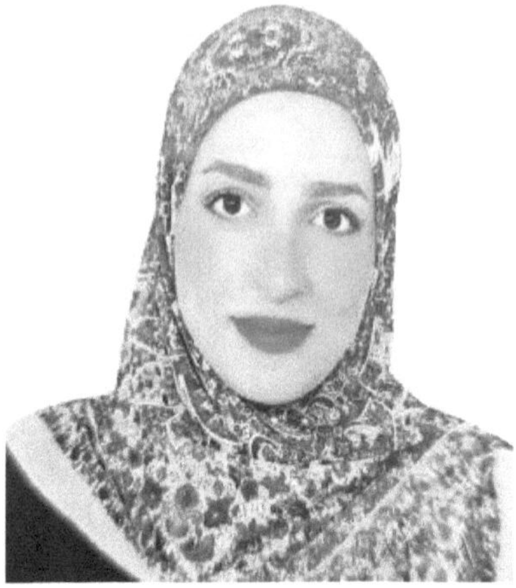

Dr. Mariam Kazim Jassab

Internal and Preventive Medicine College of Veterinary Medicine Al-Qasim Green University, Iraq

Content list

Introduction

Animal pathology is the branch of the science that is concerned with the diseases that plague animals, their causes, mechanisms and consequences of the diseases. The discipline has similarities to human pathology, but is further adjusted to non-human species. The study of the pathological changes; such as lesions or abnormal growths, enables veterinarians and other researchers to improve their ability to diagnose and treat diseases in animals, which translates into improved animal wellness and human health. Animal pathology is both a conglomeration of numerous fields including histopathology, microbiology and molecular pathology and thus provides a multi faceted method of protecting the lives of animals.

Animal physiology on the other hand deals with the study of the functioning of the body of an animal. Pathology, in its turn, explores the functional and structural expressions of disease. The two disciplines have a very close interconnection particularly because disease is a manifestation of deviation of normal physiological functions or homeostasis. This therefore means that a thorough comprehension of the fine balance of normal functioning is critical in the process of identification, diagnosis and treatment of disease-induced abnormalities.

A combination of pathological factors and physiological. Pathology is the study of the medical side of the conditions that occur in the state of disease, and physiology is the study of the biological processes and mechanisms in an organism.Pathology deals with abnormal or undesirable conditions, whereas pathophysiology addresses functional changes within an individual due to disease or pathologic states.

Johannes Müller played a key role in establishing separate physiology research from medical research in Germany during the 1830s. Davaine conducted an experiment with rabbits injected with a minute amount of putrid blood to replicate sepsis, introducing the term "ferment of putrefaction" which generated ambiguity regarding whether it referred to a microorganism similar to Pasteur's ferment or a chemical like other instances. In 1878, Koch published "Aetiology of Traumatic Infectious Diseases," a groundbreaking work establishing the causation of diseases through the injection of putrid materials into animals, according to historians.

Koch utilized bacteriology and innovative aniline dye staining techniques to identify specific bacteria for each disease. The germ theory of disease introduced the concept of a discernible cause through scientific exploration. The inception of the Pasteur Institute and Berlin Institute for Infectious Diseases in 1888 and 1891, respectively, with Pasteur and Koch as the founding directors marked the establishment of the earliest biomedical institutions. The Rockefeller Institute for Medical Research, the inaugural American biomedical establishment formed in 1901, saw Welch appointed as its scientific director, who subsequently brought in his former student, Simon Flexner, as the director of pathology and bacteriology laboratories. [4].

The Rockefeller Institute became one of the leading institutions of the field of biomedical research during the First and Second World Wars.

The 1918 influenza pandemic aroused a desperate search into efforts to determine its etiology; however, a large portion of the deaths were attributed to lobar pneumonia, which was already linked to pneumococcal invasion. In 1928, Fred Griffith, a pathologist working with the Ministry of Health in London, made a groundbreaking discovery regarding pneumococcal transformation from virulent to non-virulent forms and across different antigenic strains — resembling a species switch — aiming to unravel the specific cause of pneumonia. Findings also shocked the laboratory of the revered pneumococcal researcher, Oswald Avery in the Rockefeller Institute to the point that they could not repeat the experiment.

Mendelian genetics became a discipline during the early twentieth century and as early as 1903 the linking of Mendelian characters with chromosomes was understood, thus producing chromosomal genetics.

At the same time, the science of biochemistry started to emerge.

The majority of scientists then believed that a cell was simply a container of other chemicals and that the presence of chromosomes were the only unique structures of the cell which they believed were not present in bacterial cells.

Due to the perceived simplicity of chromosomal DNA, scientists strived to identify genes in the chromosomal proteins.

However in 1953 a breakthrough occurred as the American biologist James Watson, the British physicist Francis Crick and the British chemist Rosalind Franklin discovered the basic double-helical structure of the DNA and postulated that it must carry genetic information.

Later in the 1930s the Rockefeller Foundation launched and funded a molecular-biology research program, chaired mainly by physicist Max Delbrück at Caltech and Vanderbilt University, to explore the nature of living organisms on a fundamental level.

However, the presence of organelles in the cells was still a contentious issue due to the drawbacks of the traditional light microscopy that could not help view the organelles.

By the mid-20th century, cell biology had become an independent field of study, particularly due to cancer-research efforts of the Rockefeller Institute, which thus connected the branches of cytology and biochemistry by using the newest technologies, including ultracentrifugation and electron microscopy, to study the structure, activity and mechanism of cells.

The ethics and the science of pathology

As it concerns the study using animal models brings the issue of whether a comparative pathologist is necessary.

This is a critical aspect towards the proper characterization and validation of models that simulate human conditions in the biomedical research. There is a growing demand in universities, research foundations, and pharmaceutical companies to have animal models that help in the understanding of physiological processes about basic science as well as clinical use. Popularized models include immunodeficient, chemically induced, surgically induced and genetically engineered models based on the disease or entity of interest. One of the most commonly used ones is the genetically engineered mouse (GEM). The growth of preclinical studies and identification of biomarkers have presented a wider range of models. Histopathological evaluation is often a key aspect of translational studies in these models and majorly depends on the skills of comparative pathologists with specialized expertise and vast experience in the pathology of rodent and non-rodent models. [5-7].

This means that the number of people who have an in-depth knowledge of the unique biology of different animal species and are able to competently categorize the models who are generated and used are in high demand. Comparative pathologists, therefore, have a necessity of occupying a vital position in the validation of animal models of human disease. Comparative pathologists have a crucial role to play on research teams, in effect testing human pathological animal models, by virtue of the qualifications required to serve such teams, such as the background, expertise, experience, and skill. In addition to their usual duties as pathologists, comparative pathologists can provide expert advice in the development of animal models, test design, the correct collection of specimens and interpretation of data. Although making a thorough examination of different animal models is far beyond the capacity of this manuscript, the importance of involving a comparative pathologist and considering certain aspects of pathology at is also important various phases of translational research utilizing animal models will be discussed, with a particular emphasis on mouse models of human diseases [8,9].

Genetically Modified Models

Genetically engineered models are commonly used to study the pathophysiology of human pathways, both molecular and genetic, in an attempt to come up with effective ways of treatment or prevention.

Some of the widely used genetically engineered models (GEM) include rodents that have undergone genetic engineering to adopt features relevant to a certain human disease.

These GEM models are thoroughly evaluated in order to uncover phenotypes that are applicable to the disease being studied. Phenotyping studies of GEM models require prior planning; the research question or hypothesis determines the number of animals necessary and data analysis and interpretation.

Detailed data on the model will be mandatory, with information on the source and genetic lineage of the mice or the embryonic stem cells, any genetic alterations done to them, and special quality-control measures about genetic characteristics. Genetic alterations must be described in detail to facilitate accurate pathological evaluation and include the information about the gene of interest, the type of genetic construct that was used, the tissue specificity, the type of promoter that was used, and information on whether the model is conditional or not. The knowledge about the way of the generation and peculiarities of the model being studied is vital to the process of a pathological assessment.

The scientific literature explains different technical methods of mouse model generation. Detailed description of any conditional mutagenesis methods is necessary before subjecting the pathologist leading the research to the technology since the tissue-specific Cre technology can have its effects felt in other tissues not being targeted. The non-targeted impacts of the engineered phenotype of GEM technology can consist of changes in the usual microbiome and flora because of the antibiotic effect of tetracycline-based systems and the presence of tamoxifen in the corn oil in inducible systems. In addition, GEM models can also have unexpected phenotypes because transgenes are randomly integrated. In this regard therefore, according to the later to be discussed, any pathological assessment should have proper controls in its process in order to provide a proper interpretation of the findings [10- 13].

Genetically Modified Models

Background Strain

Genetic differences have a strong impact on the formation of animal models. When choosing a genetic background, it is critical that the comprehensive assessment of the great variety of pathological, behavioral, immunological, and physiological disparities described between inbred and outbred strains is conducted. These differences can have a significant impact on experimental results, especially with rodent models and genetically engineered models (GEMs), the background strain and substrain selection determine the expression of certain lesions as well as neoplasia.

Remarkably, variations in immunity response to pathogens evidenced in the studies of infectious diseases, and divergent susceptibility to tumour formation in the models of carcinogenesis have been attributed to specific background strains.

Furthermore, certain strains have increased resistance to tumour development whereas others have an increased predisposition to neoplasia.

Moreover, the range of tumor phenotypes realized in considered models may vary based on the genetic background of the used strain [14 -20].

On the other hand, these lesions may be misunderstood as an exemplary phenotype or they may trigger unexpected death. The comparative pathologist should have knowledge of these ubiquitous background lesions, herein referred to background lesions to be able to differentiate between them and those that are genuinely caused by genetic factors [21].

Thus, genetic background of the pathologists involved in their research requires a thorough evaluation of the genetic background including information about the particular strain of the mouse used, the substrain, the breeding lineage, and the backcross generation. Genetic variation can also be observed among members of different individuals even in inbred strains due to the divergent origination.

One must determine the exact supplier/origin of the background strain so that the precise comparisons can be made because the supplier substrains could have genetically diverged off of the original strain, and thus could potentially have an impact on the interpretation of the model [22].

The correct curbing of the model as well as accurate knowledge of the information requires application of the vendor-specific details and accurate terminology regarding the mice, genes, and any genetic modifications Guidelines for proper nomenclature can be found in this publication and other sources.

The advancement of modern models, like CRISPR, has led to advantageous variations among strains, allowing for the generation of mutations on specific genetic backgrounds [24-26].

Samples from humans and cell cultures

Xenografts of human tumor cell lines and specimens obtained from tumor patients are commonly employed in the conduct of in vivo studies pertaining to human malignancies.

The advantage of utilizing such models lies in the fact that primary samples from patients are employed, thereby directly reflecting the human disease at hand; nevertheless, the successful engraftment of these samples necessitates the utilization of animals with compromised immune systems. Several commonly utilized immunodeficient models possess severe immunocompromise and may necessitate specific housing and adherence to pathogen-free conditions due to their susceptibility [27].

Conventional specific pathogen-free (SPF) conditions may not be suitable for these background strains with severe immunocompromise. Biological materials have the potential to contain unwanted pathogens which could result in infection and spread within mice when used in experimental procedures. In some cases, these pathogens may even be transmissible to humans, as seen with lymphocytic choriomeningitis. As a result, it is crucial to rigorously test and screen cell lines and tumors to confirm they are free of infectious agents that could harm both rodents and humans, and to verify their origin from the appropriate host species [28]

Factors to be taken into account in managing one's spouse

Considerations for animal care and key factors to consider when analyzing studies include vivarium placement, animal health, cage type, bedding material, housing density, light and dark cycles, temperature, humidity levels, diet, and water quality. Changes in animal care practices and environmental factors have the ability to influence the microbiome, increase susceptibility to opportunistic infections, and potentially modify the established model phenotype [30].

The nature and the content of commercially processed diets can be very different due to the variability of ingredients and formula. Despite the fact that such diets are balanced in terms of nutritional content, they may be affected by processing methods via irradiation or autoclaving, storage, and specific feeding procedures used in the facility. These variables can influence nutrient levels, intake levels, research findings, phenotypic manifestations and general survival levels.

Overcrowding can lead to aggression-based injuries or premature death especially in male mice. Nevertheless, residential or less-dense housing might make it more difficult and add biases to the pathology testing, which would result in a single-sex study that will lead to biased results. This problem is particularly important in studies lasting many years that are dedicated to aging or survival results. It is therefore indispensable to adopt concurrent littermate controls within the same facility that experience same environmental conditions so as to gain a holistic picture of how the environment affects research models. It is imperative that both male and female subjects should be involved in research to be able to assess sex-specific reactions. [31].

Infectious organisms

Owing to introduction of SPF requirements, the cases of serious infectious agents have been reduced drastically. One must note the influence of the new agents and some commensal organisms that can be termed as permissible. The study of pathology demands understating the definite SPF circumstances and limited agents in the institution and facility. Also, one should be aware of the barriers that the facility as a whole and the individual rooms have, especially considering the model under research. The harsh infectious agents can cause deaths.

A number of the facilities utilize sentinel mice to check against pathogens and general well-being of the animals. Pathologists need to be taught the kind of barrier facilities, approved or prohibited pathogens, sentinel strains, sentinel sex and health reports as a part of the experimental setup.

Closely collaborating with the veterinary team at the facility is essential in terms of effective communication on health issues prior to death as well as any unexpected pathogen that may influence the properties of the model [31-33].

Infectious organisms

Any scientific study involves controls; hence, it ought to be infused into the experimental setup regularly. There must be both positive and negative control groups so as to facilitate the validity of results. In toxicological studies, positive controls are provided to verify the existence of a response whereas negative controls are those that are not treated and assist in creating a baseline of treatment related responses. A vehicle control is required in administering compounds or chemicals.

Similar living conditions in terms of location within the vivarium, general health condition, bedding material, housing density, lighting schedule, temperature, humidity level, diet composition as well as water source are beneficial to have concurrent controls which are littermates [17].

Although five to ten mice per group is usually the recommended number, with both sexes being represented, it is important to consider the statistical power when setting the sample size in order to ensure that the research findings can be reproducible. Addition of parallel controls when at the right age is also crucial to evaluate the phenotype since the occurrence of background lesions may change with age and thus may make interpretation of the experimental groups more difficult.

The age-related changes and disease development should be considered when studying the correlation between a particular genetic modification (GEM) and cancer. It is important to mention that malignancy can only manifest itself in old animals and primary tumors might appear in systems that have not been initially targeted. [30].

Necropsy and histopathological examination

Before a necropsy is done and tissues are collected, several issues should be put into consideration.

A standardized and systematic method based on guidelines should be embraced since it will result into increased accuracy, consistency, and value of the pathology data collected.

The objectives of the study should be outlined by the clear necropsy plan and protocol. [8].

Budgets that should be taken into account

Histopathological assessment needs adequate monetary assets and unwavering dedication in maintaining funding of the pathological end points as well as analyses. Failure to plan the requirements of pathology can have a serious adverse effect on the interpretation of final molecular and functional data, especially in long-term studies. Morphological examination is achievable in a thorough and economical manner in a case where an exclusive budget is allocated to histopathological examination.

The engagement of a pathologist in the budgetary planning procedure may save the unnecessary spending of funds and guarantee the provision of the relevant funds [30].

Considerations to make in regards to the Endpoint

The veterinary team of the facility will be necessary in the development of the clinical presentations and evaluation criteria that will significantly influence the endpoints of the study. In case of genetically engineered mouse (GEM) models, the endpoints can be selected depending on the phenotypic characteristics of the model.

The definition of the endpoint criteria is also especially significant when it comes to long-term studies or the studies that relate to aging because such studies might need extra considerations in setting the endpoints.

Cross-sectional studies also might prove beneficial in research of carcinogenesis, in which evaluation of neoplastic burden is done at specified time points. The evaluation points usually have this evaluation at fixed intervals.

Blood and Blood-Forming-Tissues

In the early discussion and planning of the necropsy procedure, a complete analysis of blood cell testing, a white-blood-cell differential, as well as serum biochemistry is suggested. These studies are meant to improve the description of phenotypes, and to aid in the research on toxicology. Control mice must be sex and age matched in order to compare appropriately as the range of controls that are provided by the testing facility might not be genetically specific or environment specific.

It is therefore recommended to experiment with five to six mice in each group with the help of proper controls to identify any aberrant or trends. Such factors as the way of euthanasia, place of collection, and blood sampling method may affect the test results. To be consistent, though, it is advisable to have consistency in terms of the collection method, the analyzers as well as the staff that will be in charge of examining the blood samples during the period of the study [33- 35].

When the various treatment groups are also taken into consideration during the blood collection, the animals will be recommended to be collected at different times so as to reduce the effect of the day-to-day variations. To ensure accurate analysis and understanding of hematologic data, consistency in the way of handling, collection time, sampling sites, methods, and the choice of special instruments is necessary to ensure that the information obtained is accurate. To achieve proper comparison between or within research studies, consistency in the site of bone marrow collection, slide preparation, and evaluation is advised [3638].

Spleen and liver are also an essential location of hematopoiesis in mice, and extramedullary hematopoiesis is induced by anemia and other diseases. In this regard, detailed hematologic examination must involve the analysis of peripheral blood, bone marrow, spleen, and liver.

It is important that positive control tissues are prepared to be optimised with antibodies.

One should also consider checking up the pertinent protocols in the immunohistochemical procedures and choosing proper primary antibodies as part of the necropsy plan, and it can also be justified to take control tissues during necropsy. This could be by collection of positive tissues expressing a given antigen, and verification of genotype and tissue expression, which are of relevance to the model. Strategic planning is hence suggested to be applied to maintain adequate collection of tissues that could be used in the future to conduct molecular tests and immunostaining. Samples should be prepared effectively in order to produce the best results. There are other sources of information on immunohistochemistry, and other publications about it [39, 40].

Extensive study of the dead specimen to do research

A necropsy is an analogous procedure of an autopsy and is performed on animals to access and extract organs and tissues after death with the specific aim of studying them. Different procedures can be used to perform a complete necropsy. The specific research goals and questions will provide the protocol to be followed; however, the common and accepted protocol is considered to follow a standard and systematic approach that is based on the well-established recommendations.

The same rules can be used with nonrodent animal models common in the academic sphere. It should be remembered that necropsy procedures can vary based on the study being conducted especially in a toxicity study that necessitates some standard operating procedures. In either case, when dealing with a new model, it is advisable to collect and assess a complete range of tissues. Evidence-based, systematic approach, depending on the needs of the study, can help to be exhaustive and contribute to the better reliability and applicability of the collected data [41-43].

To be able to separate a true phenotype and a pathology due to strain, it is necessary to examine a complete set of tissues, including the evaluation of controls that were age- and sex-matched, and with the same genetic background (ideally littermates). Animal-to-animal as well as necropsy-sequence randomisation are recommended to minimise variability and possible bias. In case of large cohorts being subjected to necropsy and tissue collection, a given number of each group must be processed on a day-to-day basis to ensure uniformity.

It is necessary to prioritize the tissue collection based on necessity and the need to conduct further testing. Although necropsy practice might be dependent on the requirements of the study, it is important to highlight that proper collection, fixation, and storage of all tissues that are to be used in the future should be done. [44-48].

As an example, the Swiss roll method can be used to make a gastrointestinal model; at the same time, separate lobes of the prostate can be isolated to make a model of the rodent prostate cancer and pathophysiology of other diseases of the male reproductive system. Similarly, whole mounts of the mamary can be used in rodent mamary models.

A uniform set of guidelines on how to trim and embed it is essential whenever conducting a necropsy to ensure consistency throughout the study. The RENI guidelines suggest the best necropsy techniques, the best way to trim the organs, the orientation of the organs and the best number of sections of organs in rodent models. Cases of detailed sets of tissues applicable to histological analysis are found in the existing literature [4951].

Ways of composition and methodology of fixation and the length of time the fixative solutions are exposed to are variables that potentially affect tissue structure and applications. The most common fixatives of aldehyde are glutaraldehyde, paraformaldehyde and formaldehyde. The most common morphological analysis is that using neutral-buffered 10 per cent formalin and freshly prepared 4 per cent paraformaldehyde.

Whole-animal perfusion, where fixative is injected directly into the body, has specific benefits in the central nervous system, and eliminates artifacts which can otherwise be seen with immersion fixation, especially when removing the brain. The whole-body perfusion can also be used to enhance fixation in other organ systems, which will provide extensive, practically artifact-free data that could finally lead to cost reductions. fixative used should depend on the type of tissue being studied.

In designing an immunohistochemical study, the Bouin fixative should be used with care due to the effects that it has on destroying antigens. The fixatives are all toxic and corrosive and explosive fixatives like Bouin containing picric acid will need special consideration and storage and handling procedures. Bouin is a fixative that fixes quickly; therefore, the tissues need to be removed immediately and washed under water to avoid over-fixing and brittle nature [52].

As fixatives, the high quality fixatives are recommended to be at least 10 times higher than the volume of tissue to reach the highest fixation rates.

Fixation needs to be conducted at room temperature, and the size of the tissue should not be exceeded to 2 to 3 mm in thickness, and 15 to 20 mm in width.

To avoid irreversible damage and artifacts in tissues, it is advisable that a consultation with the pathologist, who will examine the tissues, as well as with the laboratory that will process them, is conducted to optically select and timely fixation. [41].

Genetic engineering of models of human disease has now become a vital way of characterization through the phenotyping of the models. There are quite a number of factors that have to be considered as they may include budget constraints, the animal species to be used, and the number of animals that are needed to be used in the assessment.

Transparency is needed in the methodology because there are too many variables that may affect phenotype; therefore, it is advisable to enlist the help of a comparative pathologist when drafting a phenotyping necropsy protocol.

Academic and commercial aids exist to facilitate phenotyping pathology services and the presence of a comparative pathologist often guides or guides the consultation and assessment process of the collected tissue samples.

In order to examine the phenotypic characteristics, autopsies are conducted, also known as necropsies. Phenotypic results can be affected by numerous variables as it was mentioned before. The GM mice are normally bred on mixed genetic backgrounds followed by selective cross breeding to give desired genotypes or cross breeding with other GM lines that contain other mutations. Genetic influences of varied background and specific mutation require consideration in assessing phenotypes [20, 22].

Similarly to the conventional necropsy methods, the phenotyping necropsy and tissue acquisition protocols require a standardised method of collecting, preparing, and evaluating tissues. Preferably, it is best to take the specimen when the animal is still alive since phenotyping necropsy procedures often involves taking of images, measurements of the whole carcass and each tissue, taking of tissues in an anterior to posterior manner, and obtaining of bodily fluids and blood to undergo hematological testing as complete blood counts and serum biochemistry panels. [10, 53].

This phase of rodent subjects is called necropsy

Various deaths in embryos and postnatal mice have been reported and this has necessitated the need to carry out a thorough examination of embryos, which is usually starting at embryonic day 18 and moving backwards until the cause of embryonic or perinatal death has been established. There are resources, which provide precious information about the basic biology of embryos and methods of pathological study, used to examine them [54, 55].

Based on the anatomy and to avoid any distortion of the tissues

The careful trimming and standardization of tissues must be used in ensuring consistency of the study, elimination of the expensive artifacts and proper histological assessment. The methodology and choice of fixative to be used on tissues needs to be carefully considered to prevent tissue-specific artifacts. Special precaution must be observed with brain tissue, namely, when performing extractions out of the skull as well as fixation in the neutral buffered 10% formalin, to avoid the occurrence of dark neuron artifacts

Whole-body intravascular perfusion is the best methodology to use in order to optimally preserve morphology and minimize artifact. During the routine necropsy process, it is possible to leave the brain in the skull with the calvarium detached and immersed in a fixation solution or to leave the brain in the skull where it is then fixed, decalcified and coronal sectioned of the whole head [41].

Although different decalcification procedures are available, including those that use formic acid-based solutions, it is proposed that the fixation of bones in neutral buffered 10% formalin and subsequent decalcification with the help of a chelating agent like EDTA should be fixed on the spot. This is a method that will provide the maximum scope of histochemical and immunohistochemical special staining rather than maintaining cell morphology [37, 40, 56].

Examination and lung inflation are to be routinely done as a part of postmortem examination. This process is especially crucial with the pulmonary disease where inflation must be caused by fixation to prevent the anomalies of the process, including incomplete inflation. This may result in decreased assessment when misinterpretation of collapsed alveoli and septae is considered interstitial pneumonia. It should be watched so as not to overinflate; excessively inflate the perivascular and peribronchiolar collagen fibres might be artificially detached and a shadow of something resembling perivascular interstitial edema is created. Septal walls may also suffer such distortion making it difficult to properly determine emphysema [41, 56].

As discussed above, the inspection of the entire length of the intestine is achievable with the preparation of small and large intestinal gut roll, which usually constitute one to two slides. As much as this technique provides an in-depth evaluation of the intestinal tract, it might not be suitable in models of gastrointestinal neoplasia, as artifacts and tangental sections may generate a wrong interpretation. Some of the models should include the gastrointestinal neoplasia, in which case it is advisable to excise the whole gastrointestinal tract between the stomach and the anus, flatten it on a piece of paper to identify it, list the lesions, and take pictures of the visually abnormal regions. The gut can then be attached in the flat position and rolled or cut into representative sections and examined histopathologically. Extensive tumor lesions can be resected and fixed in a block of normal tissue at the ends, or may be cut cross sectionally to examine them.

Regardless of the specific model of neoplasia under analysis, the preparation of step and/or serial sections plan remains irreplaceable in the future with possible application of immunohistochemical and/or histochemical special staining. This step is essential in the validation of the morphology and invasion of the tumor thus proper reporting and interpretation of results obtained in the model [41, 42].

Histopathological examination involves examination of tissues under a qualified pathologist

Tissue testing using histopathology cannot be done without in the process of animal model verification and validation. The conventional standard assessment in rodent models involves a morphological descriptive assessment.

The International Harmonisation of Nomenclature and Diagnostic Criteria of Lesions in Rats and Mice (INHAND) project is a useful tool in the classification of lesions, which provides criteria to develop standards in the nomenclature of both proliferative and non-proliferative lesions in mice and rats in the toxicologic pathology.

The Mouse Models of Human Cancers of the Consortium of the National Cancer Institute have already published the comprehensive papers on pathology consensus, which defines diagnostic criteria and nomenclature of mouse models of organ-specific human cancer. They all include a close study of microanatomy in different species and create a standardised nomenclature on the different types and grades of tumours in certain anatomic systems.

Pathologists are regularly required to review and report researches in a blinded or masked way. The practice would leave them better prepared with the necessary experience, allowing the detection of missing subtle phenotypes or change and the preclusion of diagnostic drift that otherwise would have manifested due to the absence of baseline controls.

Reporting is not the only role that is performed by a pathologist. Preferably, the pathologist would work with the research team to interpret findings, deliberate on next steps, and, where justified, suggest ancillary tests based on the findings of the pathological or phenotypic observation or to perform other cohorts pathologically. Besides analysis and reporting, the pathologist is an important figure in manuscript, abstract, and grant application preparation [8, 36].

Self-determined analysis of illnesses

Care should be taken to ensure that models are not misunderstood especially since most of the murine models are genetically engineered and have been known to exhibit unique characteristics based on genetic makeup, environmental factors, and experimental factors. Regrettably, there are many examples, often in reputable journals of science, when normal tissues of rodents were misidentified and normal artifacts misinterpreted by persons lacking the long training and experience of comparative pathologists [70].

Utilizing the services of a comparative pathologist

Currently, there is a lack of a central database or repository for identifying proficient pathologists. Social media applications, including LinkedIn, can be used to establish the networking with the pathologists. The LinkedIn Comparative Pathologist Consortium serves as a social networking service and a useful tool to comparative pathologists [66, 71].

Pathophysiology: General Principles

Knowing the pathophysiology of a disease is very vital to people working in the medical field. Nuclear medicine is a field where the functional and molecular changes are studied and one must have a deep knowledge of the pathophysiologic changes of the diseases related to the field to be able to practice in this field.

Early in the late 1970s, the discipline of pathophysiology has experienced a major revolution in the new development of molecular biology and genetics. This has assisted in a better understanding of the molecular pathology of diseases. The definition of diseases by abnormalities of normal regional biochemistry has made pathophysiology a key intermediary between pathology and physiology requiring an excellent grasp of the two fields.

Pathology involves the science of disease, its causes, course, and effects especially the structural alterations that take place. This field of medicine examines the causes of diseases and their etiologies and how they present in people in order to inform treatment interventions. Pathology is needed in any field of medicine and it has extended its demands to the molecular study of organs, tissues, and body fluids.

Disease definition is complex and can be developed in different ways. Although it might be easier to define disease on a cellular and a molecular level, individual level definition is a challenge. Medical history has seen two major concepts of disease ontological and physiological. The ontological view considers disease as a self-sufficient entity with natural progression whereas the physiological view of disease describes it as an anomaly of normal physiology or biochemistry.

The majority of diseases are caused by the damage of the cell due to the inability to achieve homeostasis. The healthy operation of the human body requires homeostasis, which is the maintenance of stable conditions in the body with the help of feedback. The body has an internal environment which is mostly made of the fluids that help in supporting cellular functions that are required to sustain life. Cells are able to grow and serve their purposes effectively as long as the body organs and tissues maintain homeostasis. [71].

During birth, the genome or genotype of an individual is filled with molecular blueprints that will then be translated into cellular structure and functioning. One gene defect may produce biochemical phenotype such as a number of clinical symptoms or phenotype, a phenomenon known as pleiotropy. A disease can be clinically heterogenous, that is, caused by multiple gene abnormalities that result in the same clinical phenotype. As a result, diseases can be defined as aberrant processes and deviations of the molecular level of many biological indicators, signalling molecules and receptors [72].

Physiology is an empirical study of normal, ideal operations of the body. The science examines the mechanical, physical, biochemical, and bioelectrical processes of unconditioned people, their organs and microscopic units that make them up. It is a wide field of science that attempts to comprehend how life works, including the molecular basis of the activity of cells up to the whole organism.

Cell biology is a particular subject that explores cell structure and cell function, cell formation, cell division, cell differentiation, and cell specialization. The field defines the overall properties found in the majority of cell types as well as explains the unique properties of specialized cells that enable them to carry out particular functions. [73].

Pathophysiology is a multidisciplinary field, a combination of pathology and physiology.

It studies the abnormalities in normal mechanical, physical and biochemical functions, which occur due to or are caused by diseases, abnormal conditions or syndromes that may not meet the criteria used to determine diseases.

Molecular disease pathophysiology is now a part of contemporary pathophysiology. In 1839, Theodor Schwann demonstrated that all living organisms are composed of individual cells [74].

Changes in cellular and tissue biology, as well as functional impairments in organs and tissues, stem from cellular injury and death. Hence, grasping the structural and functional responses of cells and tissues to injurious agents, such as genetic anomalies, is crucial for comprehending the disease process. Presently, diseases are conceptualized and analyzed in molecular terms rather than merely being described in general terms of structural modifications [75].

Cell Injury

Cellular injury occurs when a cell is unable to maintain homeostasis. The reasons for cellular injury can include lack of oxygen (hypoxia), infection, or exposure to harmful chemicals. Immunological responses, genetic abnormalities, and nutritional deficiencies can also lead to cellular damage. In the case of hypoxia, energy production through glycolysis may persist, but ischemia (reduced blood supply) can limit the availability of metabolic compounds and harm tissues more rapidly than hypoxia alone. An overview of different forms of cellular injury can be found in Figure 1.

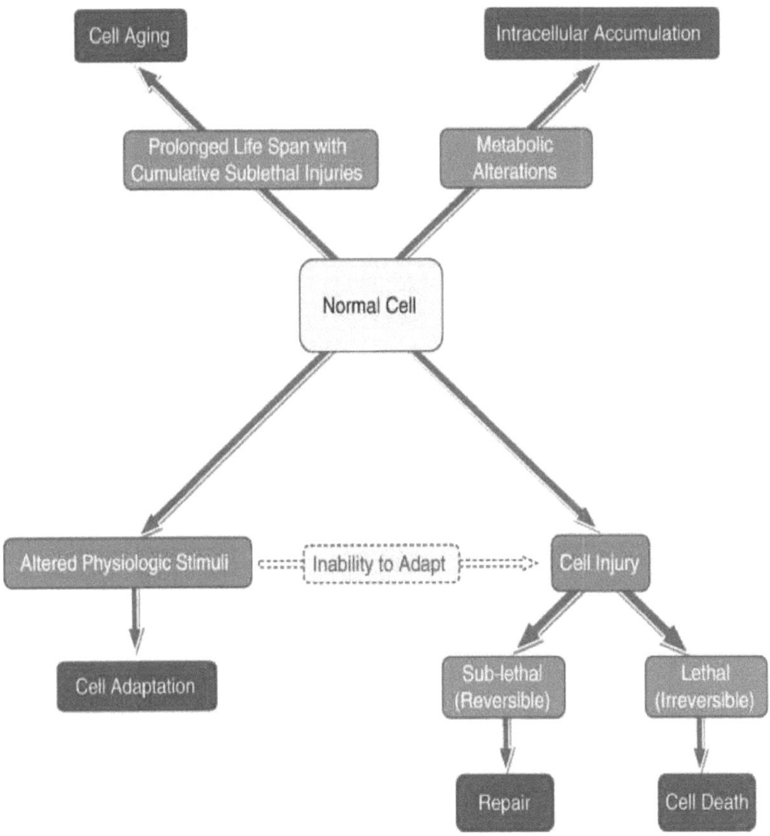

Figure (1): Cell responses to stress and injury

Biochemical Cell Injury

Irrespective of the nature of harmful agents, there are various recurring biochemical themes or mechanisms accountable for cellular injury [76]:

1. ATP depletion: The loss of ATP is a common effect of ischemic and toxic damage. This reduction leads to cellular edema, inhibition of protein synthesis, decreased transport across membranes, and membrane hyperpermeability.
2. Oxygen and oxygen-based free radicals: Ischemia causes cell injuries by limiting blood circulation and resultant oxygen shortage. Oxygen-derived free radicals are produced through radiation processes, chemicals and inflammatory processes which damage cell membranes and structures.
3. Calcium homeostasis disruption: Most of the intracellular calcium is located in the mitochondria and endoplasmic reticulum. Ischemia and some toxins cause an increase in cytoplasmic Ca 2+ levels, thus initiating the activity of different enzymes, causing intracellular damage, and raising membrane permeability.
4. Mitochondrial dysfunction: Various stimuli (e.g., high cytosolic Ca 2+ and oxidative stress) triggers the mitochondrial permeability transition (MPT) in the inner mitochondrial membrane, which finally leads to the release of cytochrome c into the cytosol. Weaknesses in membrane integrity: A variety of cellular injury, along with many bacterial toxins and viral components have deleterious influences on the integrity of membranes, thus initiating a primary disruption of membrane permeability control.

Intracellular Accumulations

Normal cells usually contain certain substances required in performing normal metabolic functions including electrolytes, lipids, glycogen, proteins, calcium, uric acid and bilirubin. Due to cell damage and metabolic imbalances, abnormal levels of a range of substances, native to the cell or exogenous, may accumulate in the cytoplasm or the nucleus on a temporal or permanent basis.

Cellular swelling that is occasioned by an excess of intracellular fluid is commonly a result of a breakdown in transport mechanisms. Dysfunctions that disturb the balance between synthesis and degradation of organic molecules including triglycerides, cholesterol, cholesterol esters, glycogen, proteins, pigments and melanin may cause unusual deposits in cells.

Dystrophic calcification tends to appear in the damaged or dead cells, whereas metastatic calcification can appear in the normal tissues due to hypercalcemia caused by the presence of increased levels of parathyroid hormone, bone tissue destruction, renal failure, and vitamin D-related diseases.

These buildups are harmful to the cells as they cause overcrowding of organelles in the cells and the formation of toxic metabolites which might or might not escape into the extracellular fluid and bloodstream.

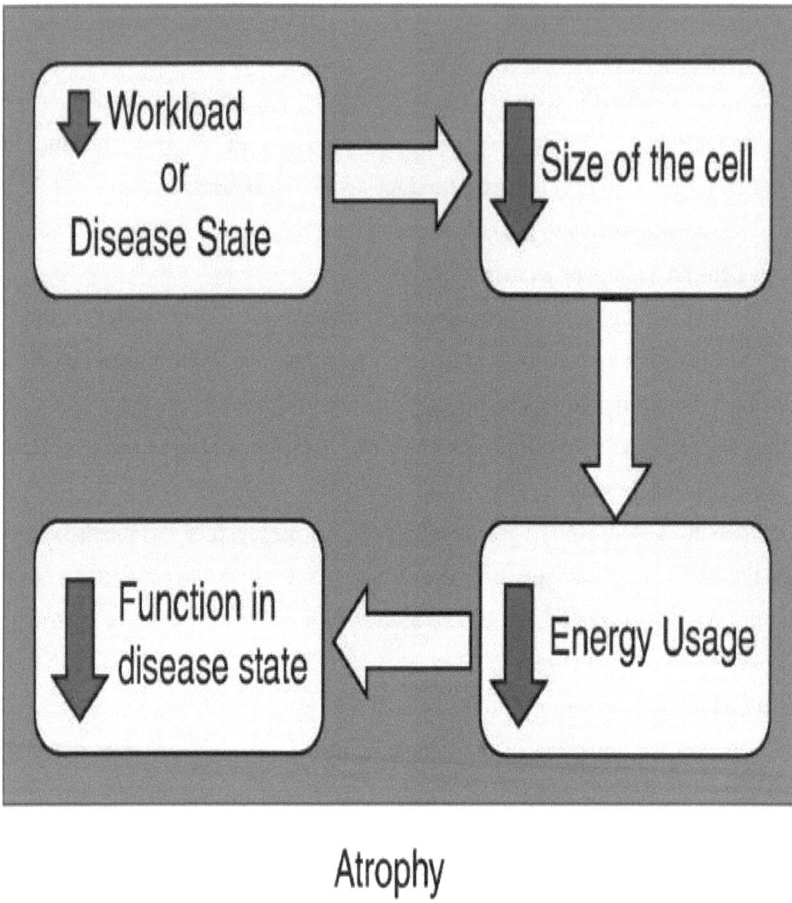

Figure (2): Atrophy

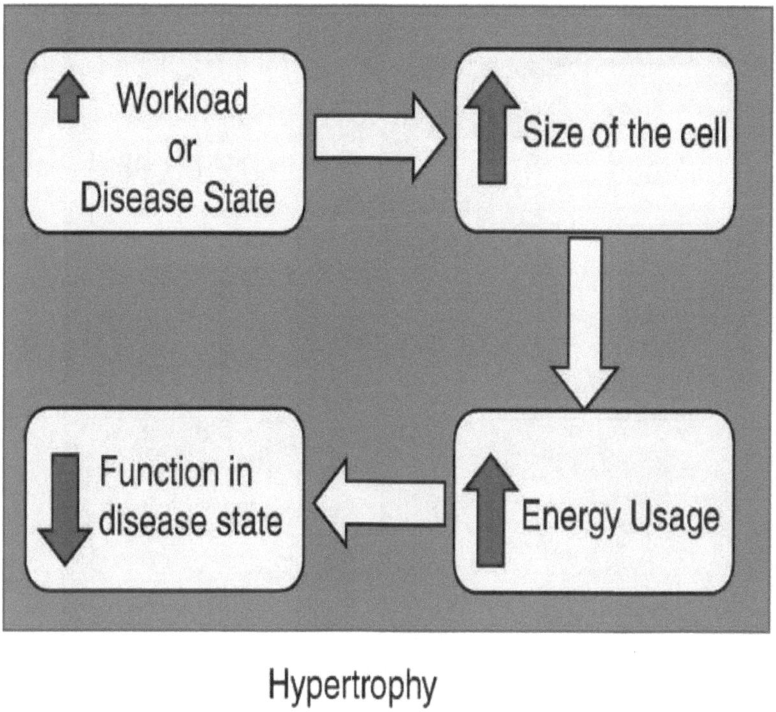

Figure (3): Hypertrophy

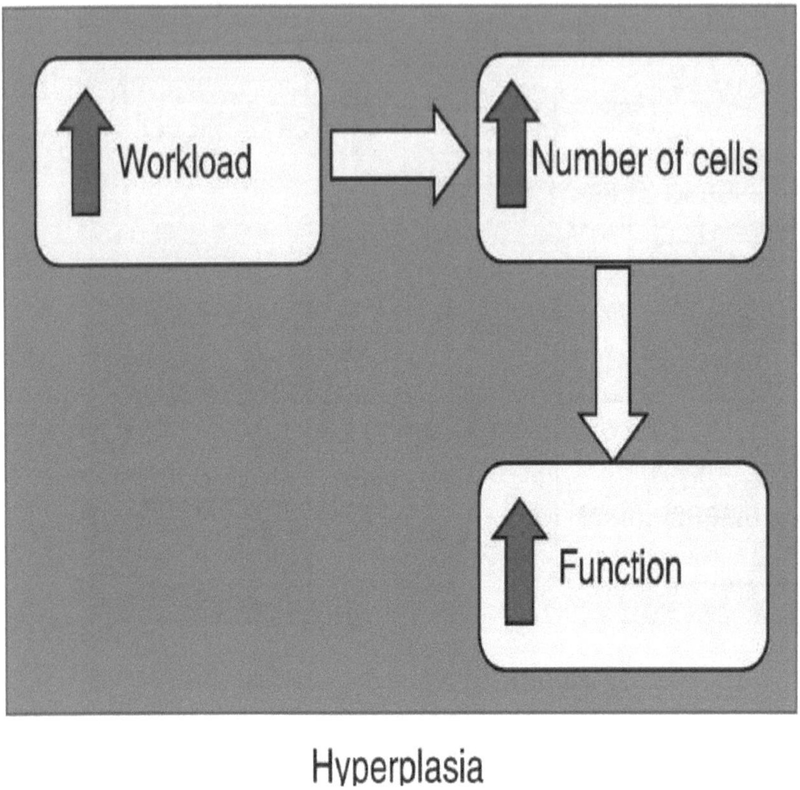

Figure (4): Hyperplasia

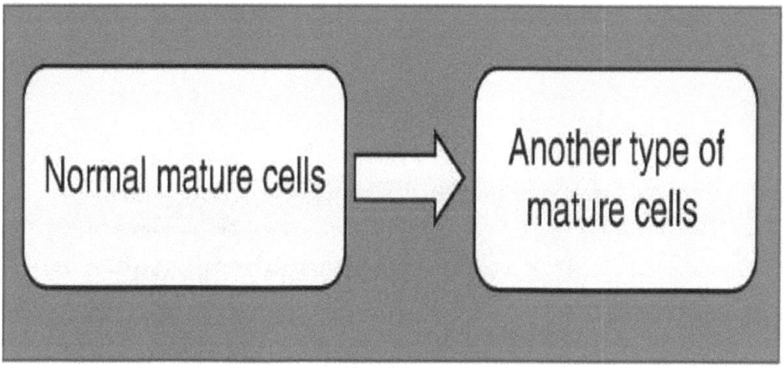

Metaplasia

Figure (5): Metaplasia

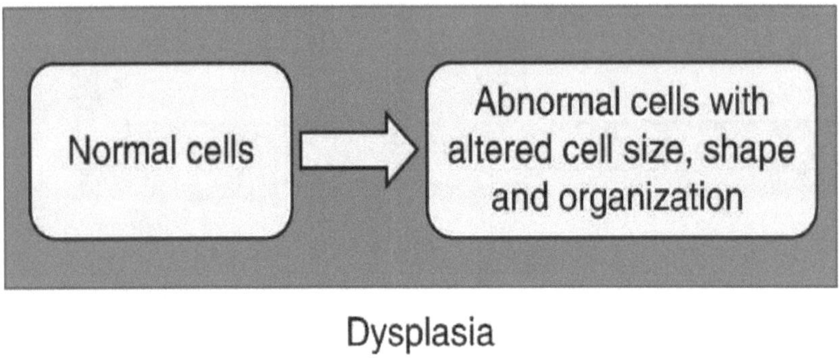

Figure (6): Dysplasia

Atrophy is a reduction in the size of the cells leading to the shrinkage of the size of a part of the body, an organ or a tissue that was previously normal, considering the age of the individual and the conditions that led to the decline. This shrinking can be caused by factors such as disuse or disease, leading to muscle atrophy.

Conversely, hypertrophy involves the non-cancerous enlargement of a tissue or organ as a result of an increase in cell size rather than quantity. An instance of this is the enlargement of myocardial muscle due to prolonged strain caused by hypertension.

Hyperplasia involves the abnormal growth or increase in the number of normal cells within an organ or tissue, usually triggered by a specific stimulus. The cells in a hyperplastic growth are still regulated by normal control mechanisms. The typical case of hyperplasia is the proliferation of the endometria caused by the increased estrogen level.

Metaplasia is a process whereby differentiated cells are converted to a different cell phenotype due to an injury or insult. This change also provides a greater resistance to the harmful effects of the offense and is normally reversible. An example of this effect is the transformation of columnar ductal cells of the salivary gland into the squamous epithelial cell under the influence of calculi. Another example is the metaplastic differentiation of glandular epithelium along the esophagus of patients who are having gastro-esophageal reflux, which is referred to as Barretts esophagus.

Dysplasia refers to the formation of abnormalities in growth or development that leads to changes in the size, shape, and structure of the adult cells or organs. It is a state that is associated with decreased mature cells alongside an increase in immature cells, which causes abnormal tissue organization. Although some of the dysplastic cells can be reversed to the original phenotype, others can be worsened and degenerate to neoplastic transformation. Unlike metaplasia, dysplasia is characterized by the retardation of the cell maturation and differentiation.

Necrosis is characterized as a type of cell death, which is uncontrolled, inflammatory and accidental

This is characterized by the swelling and permeability of cell membranes. The enzymes that are released due to necrosis break down the contents of the cells which will leak in the intercellular space, which in turn causes an inflammatory response.

The alterations in the morphology of necrotic cells can be attributed to denaturation of proteins and digestion on the cells by enzymes. Necrosis occurs in different types in different organs and tissues, the most frequent one being coagulative necrosis.

Liquefactive necrosis, however, may result secondary to ischemia or bacterial infections, with subsequent tissue softening and liquefaction being seen as a result of the breakdown of cells in hydrolases. Liquefaction takes place in the ischemic brain tissue to form cysts. Hydrolases of neutrophil lysosomes act in infected tissue, destroying both the bacteria and tissue cells in the immediate environment leading to the formation of pus. Caseous necrosis which occurs in foci of tuberculous infection is a combination of coagulative and liquefactive necrosis.

The lipase-causing necrosis leads to fat necrosis, which causes the appearance of opaque and chalky necrotic tissue which is caused by saponification of fatty acids using alkali-metal ions. The necrotic tissue and debris are later destroyed by enzymatic digestion and fragmentation or calcified.

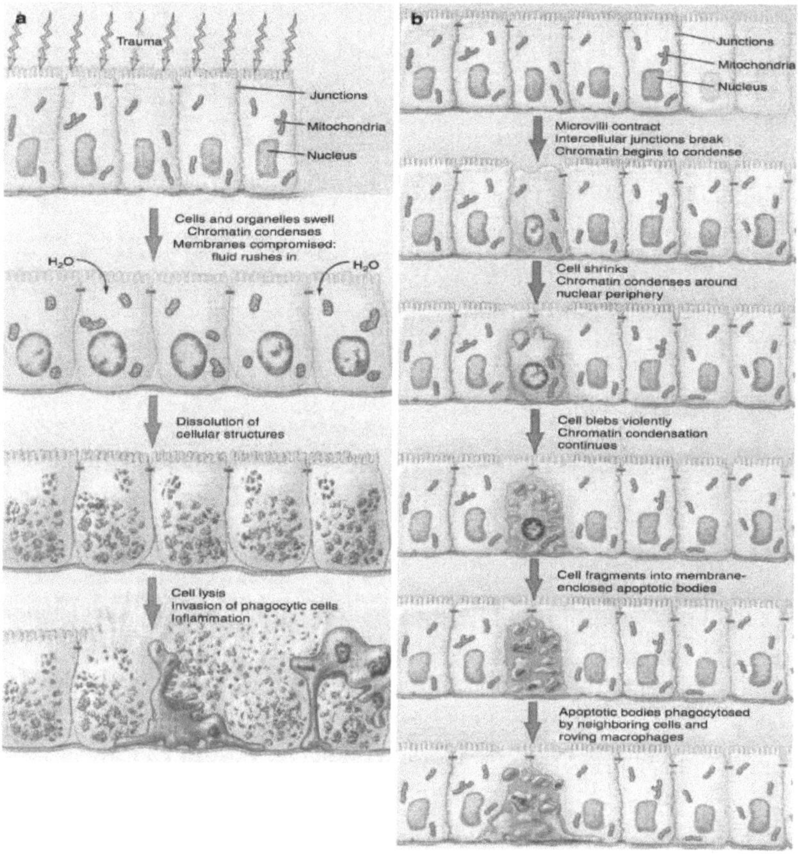

Figure 7 includes the diagrams depicting the types of cell death. Accidental cell death is achieved through cellular injury thus leading to necrosis. Necrosis is usually a cellular process and is accompanied by inflammation, which is a reaction of activated macrophages. [77]

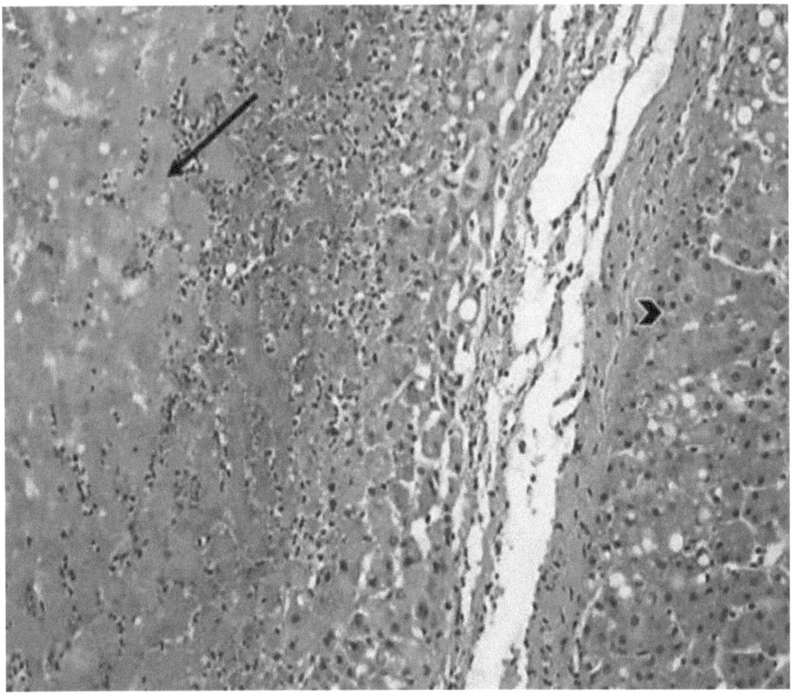

Figure 8 illustrates the occurrence of coagulative necrosis in a myocardial infarction case [77]

Apoptosis

An essential process in the embryonic stage of growth regulates the balance in the population of cells in tissues, which are a defense mechanism in immune responses and cell damage that can be caused by conditions or other adverse factors.

At later phases of the apoptotic process, executioner caspases activate a protein degradation cascade that ultimately results in the breakdown of intracellular elements, fragmentation of nuclear DNA, and cell fragmentation.

There are many morphological changes in apoptosis, such as cell contraction, condensing of chromatin and cytoplasmic protrusions called blebs and apoptotic bodies, which are then incorporated by the neighboring cells and macrophages.

In contrast to necrosis, apoptosis is a progression of controlled shrinking of the cytoplasm and nucleus, which concerns individual cells.

The apoptotic process of the mammalian cell is controlled in two major pathways, including the death-receptor pathway and the mitochondrial pathway.

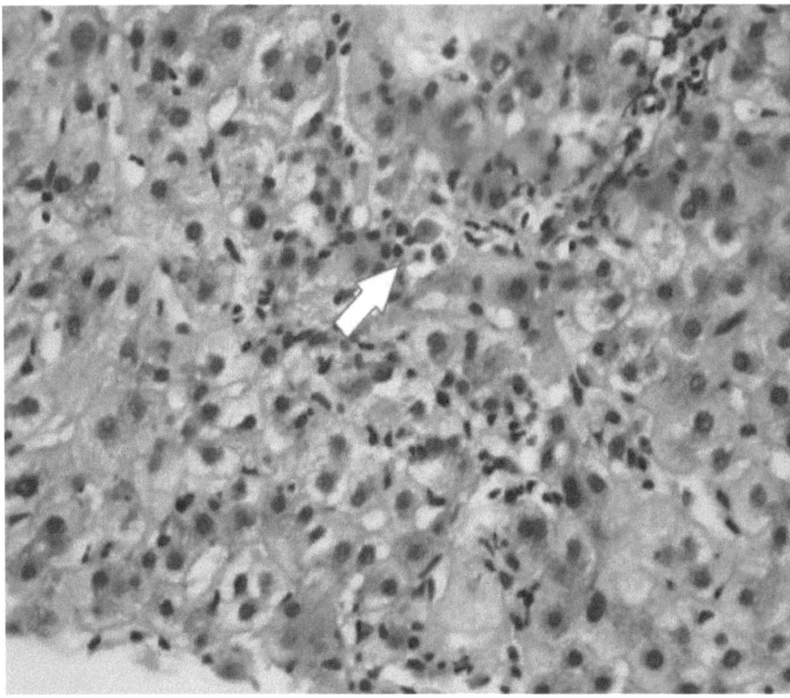

Figure 9 is the micrograph of a liver tissue sample of a patient diagnosed with hepatitis C and cirrhosis. In the biopsy, an apoptotic body, denoted by an arrow, is found in the image. [78]

Pathological conditions affecting both domestic and wild animals in the field of veterinary medicine

Veterinary pathology is a foundational aspect of veterinary medicine that specifically deals with the diagnosis and examination of diseases in animals. Veterinary pathology represents a crucial interface between clinical practice and the biological sciences with a central role to play in the clarification of etiologies, pathogenesis and clinical presentation of disease in domestic and wild animals. The field cannot be ignored in the identification of new diseases, more so those with zoonotic potential, hence improving the health status of both living and non-living organisms. Various pathologies such as infectious diseases and hereditary disorders are researched using a range of methods such as histopathology, microbiology, and molecular biology to help veterinary pathologists. In that regard, it is the role of veterinary pathology to accelerate the development of veterinary medicine as well as the improvement of animal welfare and conservation programs [79-81].

In the domestic species, veterinary pathologists are concerned with diagnosis of diseases that can befall livestock, companion animals and working animals. They include work on bacterial and viral, as well as parasitic infections, but also non-infectious diseases, like neoplasia, metabolic, and organ diseases. Such ailments cannot be effectively treated and managed without an accurate diagnosis, which can prevent the spread of infectious diseases to other animal populations and possibly to humans. Veterinary pathology in the wildlife context is important in conservation programs, where it assists in the understanding of diseases that affect the wildlife populations, particularly the one facing the risk of extinction. [82- 85].

It is the duty of the practitioners to have extensive knowledge so that they can formulate effective mechanisms of controlling diseases in the wild communities where they are aware that such diseases can have significant ecological effects. Veterinary pathologists are a key contributor to the field of public health as they are researchers in the field of zoonotic diseases- which are diseases that animals can transmit to humans.

This aspect of veterinary pathology cannot be ignored in finding possible threats to the health of the population and designing the mitigation strategies. Veterinary pathology is a field of continuous development, which is driven by the development of diagnostic methods, including molecular diagnostics and digital imaging. These inventions not only improve the accuracy but also timeliness of disease detection and therefore, the outcomes of animal health will be better. In conclusion, it is important to note that veterinary pathology is a varied and evolving discipline that must be used to protect the health and wellbeing of domestic and wildlife with serious consequences in the health of humans and preservation of the environment [86, 87].

The field of veterinary pathology does not only involve the diagnosis of diseases of individual animals, but also involves studying disease processes at the population level. This also involves the study of epidemic outbreaks in livestock which may have significant economic and public-health implications. Besides, the discipline plays a critical role in the conservation of wildlife through the advancement of the knowledge on diseases that impact the existence of wild animal population and some of them may be endangered. The pathologists in this field often work with the ecologists and conservation biologists to observe and contain diseases in the natural habitat, thus helping in the conservation of biodiversity [88].

Veterinary pathology also plays a crucial role in the treatment of chronic diseases in animals such as diabetes and arthritis, particularly because this group of diseases is becoming more common following longer animal lifespan. This trend provides evidence of the need to conduct ongoing studies on age-related diseases and create individual care plans to age animals. The discipline also faces the challenge of adapting with the diverse and, at some instances, scarce resources in the various part of globe.

Creating affordable and easy to obtain diagnostic equipment and treatments that could be universally utilized is essential to improvement of animal health on a global level. It is expected that the field of veterinary pathology will continue to evolve in the future to include additional scientific findings and technological changes to add to the knowledge and management of diseases in domestic and wild animals. [89, 90].

Veterinary pathology is an important field that facilitates the development of new therapeutic and vaccination. Veterinary pathologists can participate in pharmaceutical research, especially in immunology and oncology research through the study of animal diseases. Biomedical research often uses animal models due to their outward resemblance with humans, and veterinary pathologists make sure that these animals are provided with adequate care since there are excellent sources of essential knowledge concerning human diseases. Besides, the technological progress has influenced the sphere of veterinary pathology greatly.

Digital pathology, diagnostic and advanced imaging tools have changed the processes of diagnosing and studying animal diseases. These technologies also not only improve the accuracy of the diagnostic but also makes the detection of the diseases faster which is a prerequisite to effective disease management and control measures. Veterinary pathology is an extremely important and dynamic field that is at the crossroads of animal health, human health, and the environmental conservation. It requires a thorough knowledge of other scientific disciplines and a desire to continue learning as animal diseases and technologies to study them are ever-changing. [91].

It is a wide field that covers a lot of disciplines such as histopathology, microbiology, and molecular biology.

Veterinary pathologists make a decisive contribution in determining and describing diseases in domestic and wild animals, which is crucial to proper treatment and control of the diseases.

The field is constantly undergoing development, following the progress of medical technology and science, and thus is the foundation of the veterinary science and animal welfare.

Veterinary pathology questions the processes of disease, answers the question of their origin, course, and impact on the organism.

Pathologists rely on the study of cells, body fluids, and tissues to determine the disease and the level of health of animals.

The discipline is essential in creation of new therapies and preventive protocols that will enhance the ability of veterinary medicine to safeguard and transform the lives of animals all over the world. [92].

Disease Diagnosis in Domestic Animals

In veterinary pathology, disease diagnosis and identification of diseases in domestic animals necessitate a methodical process and therefore involves identification of a wide range of health disorders that span the infectious disease to genetic abnormalities. A set of clinical examinations, lab tests, imaging, and histopathological research are tools that are used together by pathologists to identify the nature of the disease underlying. It is an essential diagnostic method in the development of effective therapeutic programs and control of the health and productivity of domestic animals. Diagnosis is also paramount to reduce transmission of communicable diseases in the animal populations and possibly to human beings hence the multidisciplinary nature of this specialized field [93, 94].

The diagnosis of diseases affecting domestic animals is often required to have a subtle grasp of species-specific pathologies. The work of pathologists involves examination of tissue samples, laboratory diagnoses, and other diagnostics procedures aimed at revealing pathogenic agents, diagnosing organ malfunctions, and finding out genetic disorders. This all-inclusive approach will make it possible to identify diseases fast and thus provide better therapy outcomes. Furthermore, the work of veterinary pathologists is closely connected with the work of practitioners to track the progress of diseases and immunization rates and conditions, thus playing the leading role in ensuring the level of herd health and introducing biosecurity measures against the outbreak of diseases that would have a strong impact on the financial results of the agricultural and farming sectors. [93- 96].

Epidemiology and Public Health Implications

Veterinary pathology is a subset of epidemiology that involves the organized study of distribution and causes of disease-related occurrences of the animal population. This is necessary in explaining the patterns of diseases, the risk factors, and the impacts of diseases on human health particularly on zoonotic diseases.

Together with epidemiologists, veterinary pathologists study the disease outbreaks, investigate its mechanisms of transmission and develop measures of containment. It is a collaboration that cannot be done without in the timely identification and response to the emergence of infectious diseases hence protecting the animal and human communities.

In the context of the field of public health, veterinary pathology is of critical importance as it helps to understand the zoonotic diseases, which can be spread by animals to humans. This part of pathology plays a crucial role in determining the threat of potential health problems to the population, preventive strategy formulation, and policy making. Monitoring and study of animal diseases helps in increasing our knowledge of how these diseases occur, spread, and could be managed, and this would help protect human health and safety and security of food stocks. On these grounds, veterinary pathology assumes a very central position in the larger sphere of global health and epidemiology [97-99].

Role in Pharmaceutical Research and Vaccine Development

Veterinary pathology is very important in the development of pharmaceutical research and development of vaccines. The pathologists are the ones to give the fundamental details on the process of animal diseases and they are what are required in the designing of effective drugs and vaccines. Knowledge on the mechanisms of diseases and immune response would be a good resource in designing specific therapies and preventive strategies. Such contribution is especially relevant to the development of vaccines to prevent diseases of animals, and also those that can be transmitted to humans, and thus having an impact on the health of veterinary indirectly on human health.

Besides, the veterinary pathology plays a crucial role in performing safety assessment of new pharmaceuticals products to be used to ensure that they are suitable and effective in use in animals. The synergy between pharmaceutical research and veterinary pathology cannot be subjected to national interest as the development of health-related outcomes and results of medical science cannot be achieved without them [100].

They have the skill to recognize the right animal models which are close to human illnesses hence making it easier to develop new medications and treatment interventions. This interdisciplinary method does not only speed up the drug development process, but also enhances our understanding of various diseases both in the animal and human population [101].

Advancements in Diagnostic Technologies

The pathology of veterinary medicine has been transformed by the elements of diagnostic technologies, and the introduction of new methods like digital pathology has made it possible to analyse the samples of tissues with more efficiency and accuracy.

Molecular diagnostics can provide a better understanding of genetic diseases and infectious diseases and the intensiveness of the visualization of the internal anatomy and any abnormalities can be achieved with the help of the use of such methods as MRI and CT scanning.

Such technologies can improve the accuracy of the diagnosis and expedite the detection of disease thus producing a better treatment outcome [102].

Incorporation of the bioinformatics and genomic technologies in veterinary pathology has supplemented the knowledge of inherited diseases and cancer and made it possible to determine predispositions and mutations in animals to support individual and effective therapy.

Next-generation sequencing and sophisticated molecular methodologies have revolutionised the field of veterinary pathology and provided more delicate characterisation of pathogens and genetic diseases, which simplify the interventions.

Machine learning and artificial intelligence are finding their way into the diagnostic process faster and faster to quickly analyse large volumes of data, thus detecting trends and anomalies that otherwise would not be noticeable by human eyes.

These technologies facilitate the processes of diagnostics and extend forecasting abilities, thus allowing proactive and preventive medical practices in animals. [102-107].

Challenges and Future Directions in Veterinary Pathology

Despite the progress made in veterinary pathology, there are a number of challenges that have to be overcome. One of the main issues relates to the shortage of the qualified pathologists, in particular, those who have specialised knowledge of exotic and wildlife species.

Moreover, the profession should be alert to the fast changing diseases and outbreaks of new pathogens, thus requiring continuous learning and modification.

In the future, adopting improved technologies, such as artificial intelligence and precision medicine, will be indispensable.

Overcoming these issues and implementing new approaches will become the key to the future of veterinary pathology. Zoonotic diseases are likely to receive more attention in veterinary pathology in the years to come, as they have a significant implication on the health of the population. Additionally, the discipline has to deal with the issue of antibiotic resistance, thus, requiring studies to be carried out on alternative treatment and preventative measures [109-111].

There is an expected shift to the use of digital tools and data analytics in veterinary pathology, which allows conducting more advanced epidemiological studies and projects in personalised medicine. Moreover, the world has been experiencing a growing trend in global travel and trade which has necessitated the need to have international collaboration in the management of transboundary animal diseases.

The role of veterinary pathology in informing the policies and regulatory frameworks in the society will only continue to grow to make sure that the practices and animal welfare standards in the veterinary profession are in tandem with technological and scientific development [112, 113].

The way in which health and illness are understood in the field of veterinary medicine

Health and disease are the core concepts of veterinary medicine, but lack of in-depth discussion on these core concepts by the veterinary fraternity. As the level of diagnostic skills in identifying the diseases advances, it is impossible to deny the need to develop explicit definitions of disease and health since this is where the field of disease classification begins.

One of the simplistic notions of veterinary medicine that has been widely held is that health is the lack of a disease and thus brings forth a dichotomous definition [114, 115].

Pathology has continuously been a key aspect in the veterinary field. It is a well-known fact that pathologists should be competent in terms of distinguishing between health and illness in order to make relevant diagnoses. However, there are no clear definitions of these basic concepts that are regularly found and thoroughly analyzed in the field.

Regardless of the specialty field of veterinary practice, practitioners have to face the problems of health and diseases in animals every day.

Four of the 39 volumes reviewed appeared to possess more than one edition. Every issue was considered a unique handbook, and specific emphasis was devoted to any changes or additions of definitions of health or disease. There were editions with increased or modified comprehension of health and some editions with the same definitions used by a number of editions as seen in a textbook about veterinary nurses in Germany [116- 123].

Definitions of health or disease were more commonly included in non-veterinarian textbooks than in veterinarian textbooks 15 versus 7 percent respectively. Of the three textbooks on alternative veterinary medicine, which gave concrete definitions of health, all of them were presented to the lay audience, and they put special emphasis on homeopathic therapy of animals. Not only have these publications defined health in terms of alternative veterinary medicine, but also criticized what they considered to be typical medical practices. Stunningly, these publications did not have any citations and references to other sources. [124-126].

A majority of the publications merely gave one specific definition of health or disease. The only exception to this trend was that dictionaries of veterinary medicine provided alternative definitions of health. Health was hardly defined in any of the veterinary textbooks. Generally, the textbooks on pathology that were used in the mainstream did not give any clue to the definition of health and disease. Texts on pathology and internal medicine were generally divided into chapters on individual organ systems, e.g. integumentary, respiratory and digestive systems. Such textbooks were a collective work and different authors would write on diseases of a specific organ system or group of diseases. These contributions were in turn edited into book chapters by the editors [129, 130].

Health definitions encompass various classifications

Health definitions are considered as having subjective categorisation. However, this classification takes into consideration various definitions of health and diseases which vary in their complexity. The categorisation provided here is provided to give the study an organisational structure, and not necessarily a conclusive utterance to the varying points of view on the subject.

Health as normality

The definition of health and disease based on the normality or abnormality is commonplace. However, historical definitions that have seen health as normality have been quite narrow in definition and have been frequently fragmented. However, it should be noted that this definition refers to clinical health, which is based on the assumption of normality. Similarly, the disease definition of John Webster highlights how disease is related to a normal condition and how anything out of the normalcy is illness. To gain insight into the variation in normal health, Webster underlines the necessity to gain clinical experience in using healthy animals. The authors however acknowledge the fact that there are different definitions of health, without taking a firm stand in that regard [133, 134].

The use of the term disease as not at ease makes a point to their etymological definition of the term in that animal ill-health is disease. In addition, the authors suggest that the elements of biological functioning should be incorporated into the normality-based definition of health to underscore the importance of structural integrity and functional abilities in defining health other than a simplistic concept of normality. [135, 136].

Health can be viewed as a physiological state

They hypothesized that disease can be found as a form of aberrant or dysfunctional physiology, in their comparative pathology textbook. They also suggest that disease in the end, refers to structural or functional changes in the cellular elements that form the entire living organism, which forms a major idea in the discipline of pathology [137].

Another similar definition of disease is also given, which is states of the dysfunction of the normal activity of the body. According to them, disease is a change of condition of the body or its organs, and causes breaks or disturbances of normal bodily activities [138].

Veterinary pathology is something introduced as abnormal biology in a generalized perspective and it focuses on the lesion and abnormality of both structure and function that takes place in the body [139].

Maintaining a state of equilibrium in the body known as homeostasis

The homeostasis concept of health has been known since long enough and it serves as a common platform of understanding health and illness. Homeostasis refers to the fine balance that is maintained within an organism, and its physiological processes, where sickness can arise out of a disturbance of normal body functions brought about by factors such as the structure of the organism, vulnerability to disease and external conditions such as infectious pathogens, toxins and environmental conditions.

Homeostasis is so ingrained in the science of physiology that it is not just a descriptive device that explains the physiological processes but a basic law, just like evolution, that is viewed as a natural law and not a hypothetical concept [139].

Health as homeostasis is often stressed in the field of veterinary homeopathy, and the aspect of health is often discussed as a manifestation of the holistic nature of homeopathy as opposed to the conventional approach to medicine. An example is Christopher Day, who lays stress on the need to achieve harmony between mind, body, and environment to induce a state of overall health and well-being.

Health in a holistic context has been viewed as the unity of mind and body in regard to the surrounding environment. Disease is understood as a state of imbalance of either the organism or the organism and the external environment in form of physical or psychological discomfort.

Through the traditional medical system where diseases are characterized by signs and symptoms, the medical system of holistic medicine views these signs and symptoms as the reactions to the internal imbalance that has been created by external forces that disorient the body [125].

Homeopathy definitions are normally defined as being holistic and based on the belief that health is reliant on homeostasis. However, the fact that the principle of homeostasis is naturally consistent with the practice of homeopathic medicine is not substantiated, as the role of homeostasis in the definition of health is also acknowledged by conventional texts on veterinary medicine. [140, 141].

Health encompasses both physical and mental well-being

One notable exception is Martin and his colleagues, who reference the World Health Organization's definition of health as "a state of complete physical, mental, and spiritual well-being", but also emphasize the importance of productivity in farm animals.

A health definition that focuses solely on physical and psychological well-being may not align with the overall objectives of livestock production.

Similar viewpoints are expressed in the veterinary dictionary by Blood and Studdert, who define health as a state of physical and psychological well-being and of productivity including reproduction.

There may not be an immediate conflict between well-being and productivity, but it raises questions about prioritizing these aspects when they are at odds [141-144]

The concept of health encompasses various aspects, such as productivity and reproduction

The concept that animal health is directly linked to productivity is not widely seen in the literature, although it is referenced by C. S. G. Grunsell in Black's veterinary dictionary. According to this source, health is increasingly being recognized as a condition of optimal economic performance.

Although it is not common to equate health with productivity alone, several authors do incorporate aspects of reproduction and productivity in their definitions of health in farm animals. For example, Aspinall argues that a healthy animal will exhibit normal growth, reproduction, and behavior consistent with its species and breed.

In the text "Veterinary Medicine: A Textbook of the Diseases of Cattle, Sheep, Pigs, Goats & Horses," it is contended that disease has traditionally been defined as a deviation from normal structure or function, but now also includes subclinical conditions. Disease is described as encompassing a failure to meet expected nutritional and environmental standards, as well as the presence of disqualifying chemical residues in animal products.

Sainsbury extends the concept of health beyond the animal's subjective health state by arguing that medication for disease control does not truly promote health, even if the animal appears healthy [145- 147].

Health and disease were seldom explicitly defined in textbooks on veterinary medicine. This lack of clear terminology can be explained by the fact that the main theme of these writings was the description of diseases, their cause, and their effects instead of covering the fundamental ideas of health and illness.

Multiplicity of aspects of health definitions is often reflected in the textbooks, thus leaving some confusion over the key concept of health in any given book. As stated when an explicit definition of health is provided, it is normally given without giving reference to pre-existing definitions of health and this suggests that the authors are giving more emphasis to the overall theme of the text rather than speculative philosophical discussions on health.

The question of animal welfare appeared in the vet texts that were reviewed in this research conspicuously and this may indicate that the authors were usually not reliant on each other in relation to their views on health and disease. However, some exceptions were seen in the veterinary homeopathy literature, where the authors condemned the traditional veterinary medicine as using an erroneous form of health definitions, which they believed were entirely mechanistic in nature.

Homeopathic definitions of health were more focused on the idea of a holistic approach and focused on the argument that health was reliant on homeostasis.

Homeopathy and veterinary medicine have some common concepts of health, but the focus on the homeostasis does not necessarily mean the adherence to the philosophy of homeopathy. This observation suggests that the theoretical basis of the definition of health is not necessarily the basis on which the approach is adopted in the practice of veterinary practice.

The study of the health concept would have a positive contribution likely to the veterinary medicine when done more exhaustively. A veterinarian will be the person who will not think about the concept of health risk because he would be an equivalent of an animal mechanic, just by diagnosing the ailment of his animal and providing him with the a priori solution. Better definitions of health and disease would enhance the delivery of the zoonotic threat to the people and make the discussion of animal welfare more relevant through the creation of a common understanding of these basic constructs. [142-146].

The Impact on Hematobiochemical Parameters in Creole Goats

In spite of the above adaptations, extreme environmental occurrences can disrupt the internal homeostasis of these organisms, which is reflected in the alterations in their hematological and biochemical conditions which can influence the general well-being and the productivity.

Moreover, seasonal changes in forage supply and heat stress are likely to alter the levels of blood metabolites and immune cells in goats, and, therefore, affect their nutritional condition and adaptation ability [147-150].

Previous studies have clearly indicated the importance of diet in goat physiology as they have explained the dietary composition and strategic forage supplementation effects on vital hematological parameters.

Indicatively, an experiment in Ecuador showed that adding to the diets of Creole goats enhanced their immune system as manifested by a high number of leukocytes.

However, the impact of certain nutritional interventions on Andean adapted goats has not been studied adequately [151].

Past studies have determined that the linear mixed models (LMMs) are effective in longitudinal data analysis in ruminants to give detailed information on how the environment and nutrition affect physiological changes. [**152**].

Evaluation of Model Fit

The analysis will involve model comparison, with and without interaction, by the Akaike Information Criterion (AIC) and Bayesian Information Criterion (BIC), and hence, trade-off between parsimony and precision.

The model of fitting blood parameters

The results of both the ALT and ALP models were similar but the ALP model had a significant level of dispersion as a residual thus reducing its reliability. The model showed no higher efficacy even though it is more complex. The analysis of random-effects showed that ALP showed more inter-individual variability than the ALB and TP models, which were more consistent.

Testing the marginal hypotheses pertaining to fixed effects

It was found that the model reliability was dependent on the kind of parameters used hence showing differences in biological strength and susceptibility to unknown variables. Those parameters that had the least intra-individual variability including albumin (ALB) and red blood cell indices resulted in the strongest fits, indicating that they are reliable as useful prognostic indicators in high-altitude settings.

On the other hand, models that included immunological parameters (whole blood cell count, white blood cell percentage) had lower predictive strength, which could be explained by high inter-individual variability, or more importantly missing important covariates, including parasite load or vaccination history. This highlights the need to include more specific immunological biomarkers and use multivariate methods that have the ability to capture the complexity of the immune system.

The sufficiency of the fit does not just rely on the statistical method to be used, but on the biological characteristics of each variable and its interaction with the environment. Mixed models have been useful in hierarchical and repeated reporting of both fixed and random effects, and thus it has been invaluable in modeling animal husbandry.

The emergence of mixed models has made it easier to differentiate between the fixed and random effects in the hierarchical and repeated structures and this is a crucial factor in zootechnical studies. [150- **160**].

Analysis of Marginal Hypothesis Tests for Fixed Effects

These complex reactions demonstrate the changes in homeostasis caused by the environmental factors and diet, therefore, emphasizing the long-established physiological plasticity of the small ruminants to the climate and nutritional shifts.

These factors are incorporated in holistic models to use a rigorous and detail approach to analyze physiological variables in so far as various production environments are concerned.

This shows that the interaction of ecological and operational elements was to be considered when evaluating zootechnical information [161, 162].

Comparison of averages as per season of the year, the diet, and the time of sampling.

The analysis of Biochemical parameters will be done in the following manner:

(a) Biochemical parameters.

• Urea levels (mg/dl): Blood urea nitrogen (BUN) levels were significantly greater in the rainy season ($p < 0.001$) and this has been observed before by other researchers who have recorded seasonal changes in this metabolic parameter.

Total protein concentrations (g/dL): This trend is consistent with results showing the highest TP values in summer (68.75 -1 dL) and the lowest values in winter (p -1), which reveals the interrelation between reproductive physiology and seasonality.

The insignificant differences between the extensive and semi-intensive systems regarding the levels of TP suggest that the climate can be a stronger determinant of TP levels in the high-Andean environment than the moderate degrees of dietary change, which is confirmed by previous studies.

However, other studies have indicated that TP levels are influenced by physiological and genetic factors [161 -168].

The research carried out in Turkey during peripartum period found homogenous levels of TP in the range of 3.5–13 /dL, which indicates the existence of stable homeostatic mechanisms [169, 170].

The study conducted before has also indicated high levels of albumin in the rainy season. Their intricate interplay of particular elements is what leads to the alterations in albumin, and thus, the nature of the protein metabolism is dynamic, as it responds to the changes in the environment and time of the year [171-173].

Other studies show the decrease of the levels of albumin following the supplementation of the Moringa oleifera, but dietary intervention had no apparent influence on albumin levels in the current case. Furthermore, age also proved to be an important determinant of albumin levels, which indicates a complicated interaction of factors.

There was no seasonal difference in dietary alkaline phosphatase concentrations, but a large difference in dietary concentrations with higher concentrations in specific feeding groups which could be linked to the increased osteogenic activity of younger animals.

The association of bone metabolism and alkaline phosphatase was supported with the high level of values observed in certain diet and sampling groups, which may indicate that nutrition had a potential to promote osteoblastic activity. It was also observed that age might have had a role to play in alkaline phosphatase regulation with a higher degree of concentration in adults compared to younger subjects.

The effects of the dietary factors on the level of alanine aminotransferase were not statistically significant, however, the differences between the seasons and the dietary treatments were observed in the data.

This outcome is consistent with other previous research that indicates that the activity of alanine aminotransferase is possibly related to change in diet and age also plays a role in the process. The paper also highlights the importance of understanding the impact of diet and age on enzyme activity of the liver in the general health of the animal [174 -176].

There was a significant increase in the count of white blood cells during the dry season ($p < 0.05$) as an immune reaction to environmental stressors caused by the environment.

The highest count of white blood cells was found during the dry season in the animals which received diet D2 and model M3 albeit with no significant differences in other cases, maybe because of increased immune challenges necessitated by heat stress. Several studies have demonstrated that age and breed affect the concentrations of the white blood cells in the blood of the goats; age variations are however mixed with one study indicating that adult Borno White goats and female kids have high concentrations of the white blood cells in their blood. [177-180].

In some studies, seasonal changes in neutrophils were reported and thus highlighting the effects of environmental factors. Differences in values of neutrophils dependent on breed and gender were also detected and age can also be a factor leading to the differences. The relations between the breed and the environment were mentioned as possible determinants of neutrophil values [180-186].

There was a seasonal oscillation in the hemoglobin concentrations whereby high concentrations were during rainy season compared to dry season, and this indicates a better oxygenation. The hemoglobin levels decreased progressively between M1 and M3 with varying values of hemoglobin levels being recorded under different dietary and environmental conditions. Differences in adaptation among various breeds were found to be genetic, and they were believed to have contributed to the level of hemoglobin [187].

There was a significant difference in the mean corpuscular volume (MCV) of season with higher values in the dry season and no apparent change in response to diet type. The effect of interaction also shows that MCV is sensitive to seasonal conditions, which may have a physiological interaction [188-191].

Although the percentage of lymphocytes was stable with regard to seasons and diets, the percentage of lymphocytes was similar. Similar results have also been obtained, some studies showing no differences in the proportions of lymphocytes according to treatments or physiological conditions whereas others have found that there is seasonal stability or variability depending on diet and environment [192-195].

Past studies have shown that there is a relationship between the weight and the amount of energy being consumed, and the weight loss is often regarded as a result of the heat stress and the decrease in the consumption, and then the ensuing compensatory growth after weaning. [196-198].

Explaining the pathophysiology of disease among East Friesian sheep through organoid modeling

Inflammatory bowel disease (IBD) is a continuum of bowel diseases, which presents a high risk in the health and survival of large animals due to chronic inflammation. Intestinal tissues of humans and animals are characterized by a high variety of cell types.

However, in the course of IBD development, the cellular structure is disturbed, and functional deficiencies and intercellular communication disorders emerge, which leads to the breakage of the intestinal barrier and disorder in the work of the immune system, further increasing the inflammation [197, 198].

Regardless of the effectiveness of existing treatment, there is a significant difference in individual responses to it due to the heterogeneity of IBD, which leads to the emergence of drug tolerance in certain patients. This, therefore, stems a dire need to come up with novel therapeutic approaches based on a greater understanding of the underlying pathophysiology.

Animal models in the past have been the main tool of studying the mechanisms of IBD and testing the efficacy of therapeutic interventions, which provides a detailed understanding of the relevant biological processes. Nevertheless, the weaknesses of humanization, interspecies physiological variability, and high-cost of such models have hampered their extensive use in mass drug testing [199-202].

Such organoids recapitulate the regenerative functions apparent in intestinal tissues, where tissue-resident adult stem cells (ASCs), are necessary in maintaining intestinal architecture and functions [203206].

Organoids are complex three-dimensional (3D) simulations of particular tissues that are grown in vitro. The use of 3D cell-culture system has a significant potential due to its ability to recreate the complicated cellular conditions.

Exploration of bovine small intestinal crypts in a 3-D culture growth factor offers worthwhile information that can further the study of organoids [212]. In our current research, organoids based on the ileal epithelium of East Friesian sheep were formed with the focus on main locations of intestinal infection.

The studies of RNA-seq samples can provide insights into the genetic makeup of these organoids, and the efficient creation of long-term cryopreservation and storage guidelines overcomes the need to use living animals in the experiments.

The inflammatory mediators, which include interleukin-1 0 (IL-1) and TNF-0 6 (tumor necrosis factor-0) are significantly increased in inflammatory bowel disease (IBD) [213]. IL -1b is a key mediator of host defense to infection and injury [214], secreted mainly by immune cells, including the macrophages in the form of 31 kDa precursor triggered by PAMP/DAMP signalling [215]. Despite there being an understanding of its activation and secretion pathways, the mechanisms that define the specific processes are not fully understood. As such, we aim to create an IL -1 -induced model of inflammation using intestinal organoids of East Friesian sheep to clarify the pathogenic processes.

The progressive rise in transepithelial permeability of paracellular markers over time after a concentration of 30 □ngml -1 IL -1b, in the range of biologically relevant doses, indicates a strong inflammatory response. The results provide useful information in order to reduce the parameters of the IL-1b concentration in our experimental set-up [216].

Extraction of Crypts from the Intestines of East Friesian Sheep

The epithelial surfaces were then exposed with aseptic equipment and a longitudinal incision was done on the ileum. To remove the digesta, the luminal surfaces were washed with DPBS before placing them on sterile Petri dishes.

This process produced a tissue pellet with a layer of mucus on it and this was carefully removed alongside the supernatant.

The tissue was then reconstituted in DPBS containing Gen -2.7 and P/S-1 and centrifugation, aspiration, and reconstitution again done till there was no mucus layer left on the tissue pellet [**217**].

The cultivation of intestinal organoids derived from East Friesian sheep

In such circumstances, crypts enclosed and intestinal systems developed within 24 hours whereas budding structures developed within day 4.

The previous studies have revealed that, IGF-1, which is rich in human plasma, is capable of inducing crypt growth in murine models.

When the culture was initiated there was found to be closing of the apex of the crypts of an apical region, which indicated growth of the area and development of enteroid-like structures whose central lumens.

Electron microscopy showed that there was progressive growth of the size of organoids with time.

Further passaging of the organoids produced normal growth and retained the ability to continue with the proliferation of the structures.

ImageJ software analysis revealed that there was a considerable growth in the area of the organoids with the length of culture.

In addition, the proliferating rate of organoids was seen to be exponential with duration of seven days to be noted which highlights the positive influence of the duration that the culture is in. While the germination rate decreased after the third generation, overall growth of the organoids remained steady [218-221].

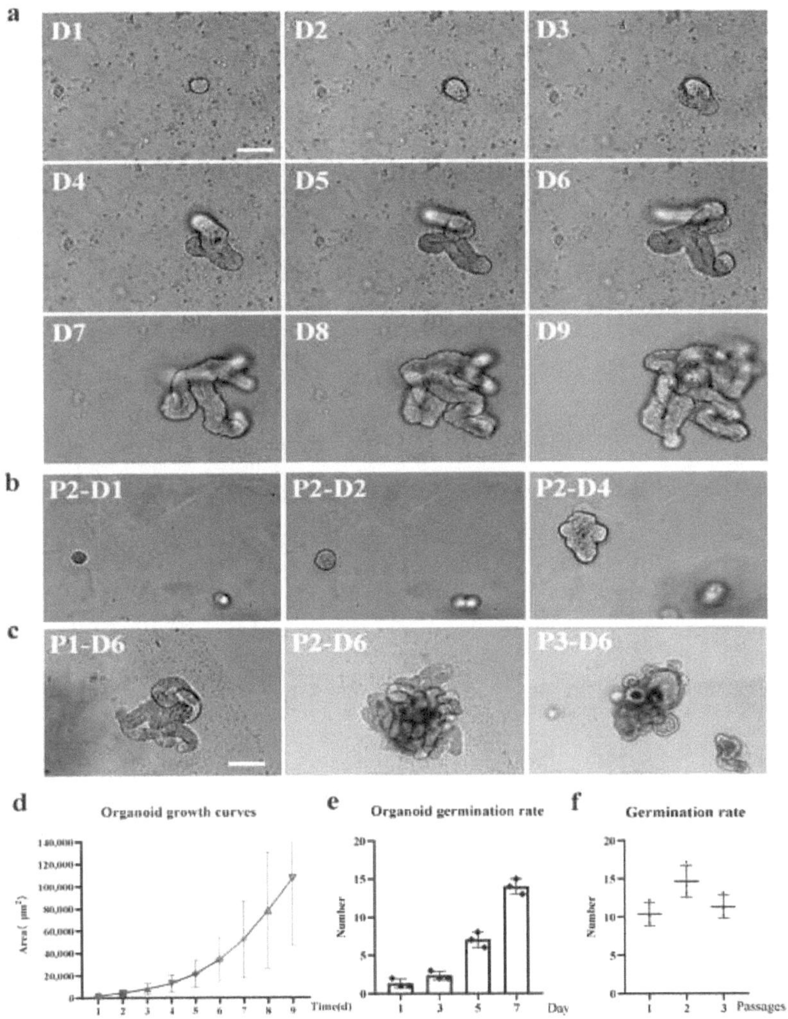

Figure 10 displays the progression of sheep enteroids cultured in an Intesticult medium on their own.

The Development of In Vitro Disease Models Using Intestinal Organoids

The markers specific to intestinal epithelial cells were detected in the organoids, thus confirming their classification as intestinal organoids (Figure 11a).

Villin, a protein that binds to actin and is unique to epithelial cells, was present in ileal organoids cultured for 7 days, and its expression decreased following treatment, affirming the accuracy of the disease model's phenotypic response (Figure 11c).

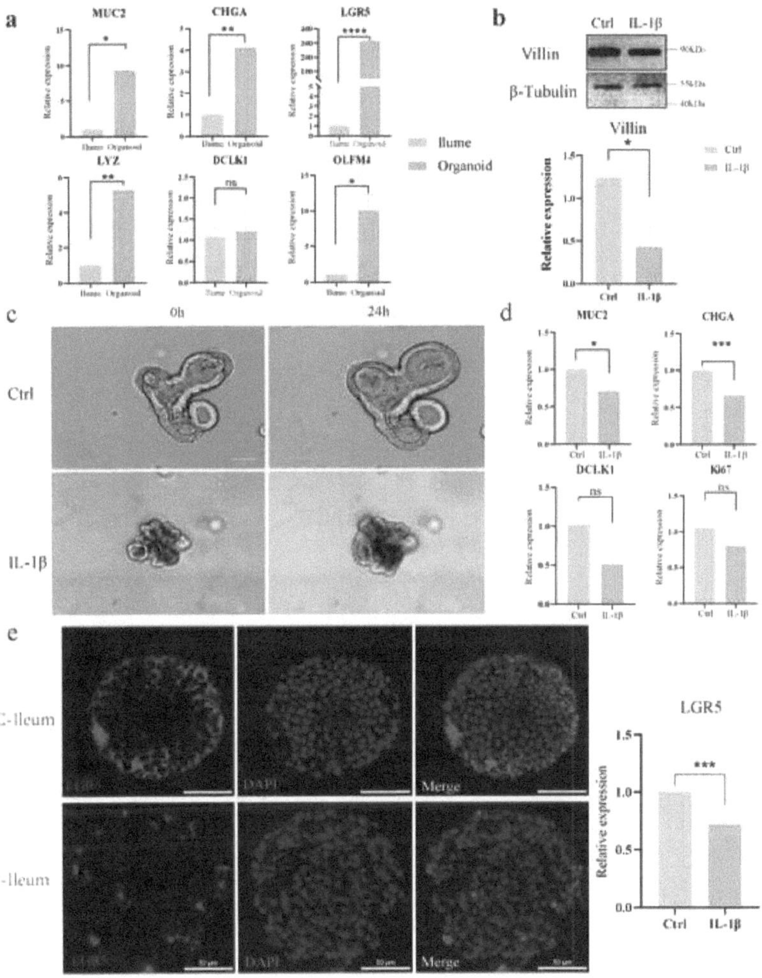

Figure 11 presents a comparative analysis of the ileum tissue and ileum-derived organoids obtained from East Friesian sheep.

β-catenin, a critical element of the adherens junction complex, collaborates with E-cadherin and α-catenin to preserve cellular adhesion and tissue structure by regulating cell proliferation and intercellular cohesion

Ki67, a marker of proliferation, along with β-catenin, was observed in both the control and IL-1β treatment groups (Figure 12a). The research authors conducted the immunofluorescence staining and quantitative analysis to investigate the expression of TNF-a in the interest of ileal organoids under diverse treatment conditions.

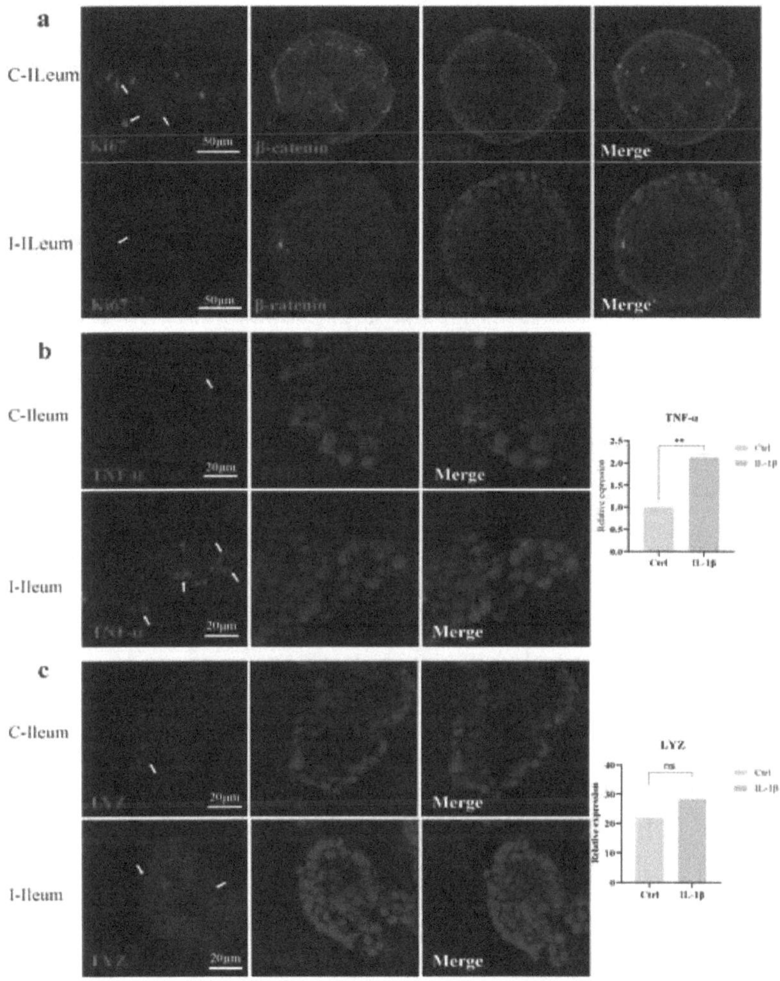

Figure 12 shows the combined results of immunofluorescence and quantitative PCR measurements in ileum organoid of East Friesian sheep.

Gene expressionin intestinal organoids after treatment with IL -1 -b was analyzed and distinct differences could be seen compared to the control. Using a principal component analysis, it was clear that there was a significant distance between the two groups in view of global gene expression patterns. There were 763 differentially expressed genes (DEGs), including 394 unique genes in the control group, 369 unique genes in the IL -1B group, and 11,445 genes expressed in both groups.

In these DEGs, 147 and 29 genes were up and down-regulated respectively in the IL-1b group. It was interesting to note that there were vast differences in the expression levels of these DEGs between the groups. Additional enrichment analysis with Gene Ontology showed that there are important biological processes related to the DEGs.

The current economic climate is not favorable to new investment activities. Assessment of affiliated risks before making any financial decision should be done with meticulousness. Moreover, the market dynamics should include the contribution of the external determinants. It is also recommended that the investment portfolio should be diversified to limit the potential losses. The achievement of long-term fiscal goals cannot be achieved without proper financial planning. A constant check on the market trend and keeping in touch with economic trends is a precondition to success in the financial markets.

The growth can only be sustained by the implementation of a well-conceived investment strategy. Exhaustive research and seeking advice of financial professionals can be of help in making an entry into the complexity of the financial market. Adjusting to the market and adjusting investment policies to suit the market changes is essential to maximize returns. The financial success that comes after the long term requires patience, hard work and flexible decision-making. Professional advice is recommended to face the complicated economic situations. Caution that is upheld in relation to market trends and economic signals can guide investment choices. The diversification is an essential aspect of effective risk management in the investing sphere. A careful study of the market conditions is unavoidable prior to making an investment decision. Monitoring the progress and making the needed changes to the investment performance is also imperative. Calculated risks are potentially more profitable to undertake; however, it is essential to analyze possible pitfalls. The need to develop a sound financial base requires a combination of sound decision making and planning. It is important to be updated on the current trends and economic activities so that informed decisions can be made in regard to investment. Conducting consultation with the experienced professionals may help guide the investment strategies towards the best financial results. Investing takes time to be successful comprehensive understanding of market dynamics and the ability to adapt to changing conditions.

On the other hand, organoids generated by the LGR5+ stem cells have the potential of autonomous organ formation that is similar to primary functions of intestinal tissue, polarized epithelial cells, contact with the extracellular environment, and multicellular populations.

The morphological and inflammatory changes in organoids exposed to IL 1b were severe, including loss of organ size, loss of the ability to form buds, and release of inflammatory mediators. After exposure to the factors of inflammation, the organoids developed within 34 days after the passage, morphological alterations, reduction in overall size, and the appearance of apoptosis in the intermediate cells.

Intestinal inflammatory models induced by inflammatory factors showed a marked increase in the activation of essential inflammatory signaling pathways, including NF- κB, TNF and IL- 17. This was observed by the increase in the expression of TNF signaling pathway downstream mediators such as TRADD and FADD which in turn initiated the apoptosis-related proteins, such as caspase-3, with IL-1b.

Exposure of IL-1b generated apparent morphological, apoptotic, and increased production of inflammatory cytokines (IL-8, CCL20, CXCL5) by MyD88TRAF6 signaling pathway.

These results support the importance of sheep intestinal organoids as powerful tools of translational studies.

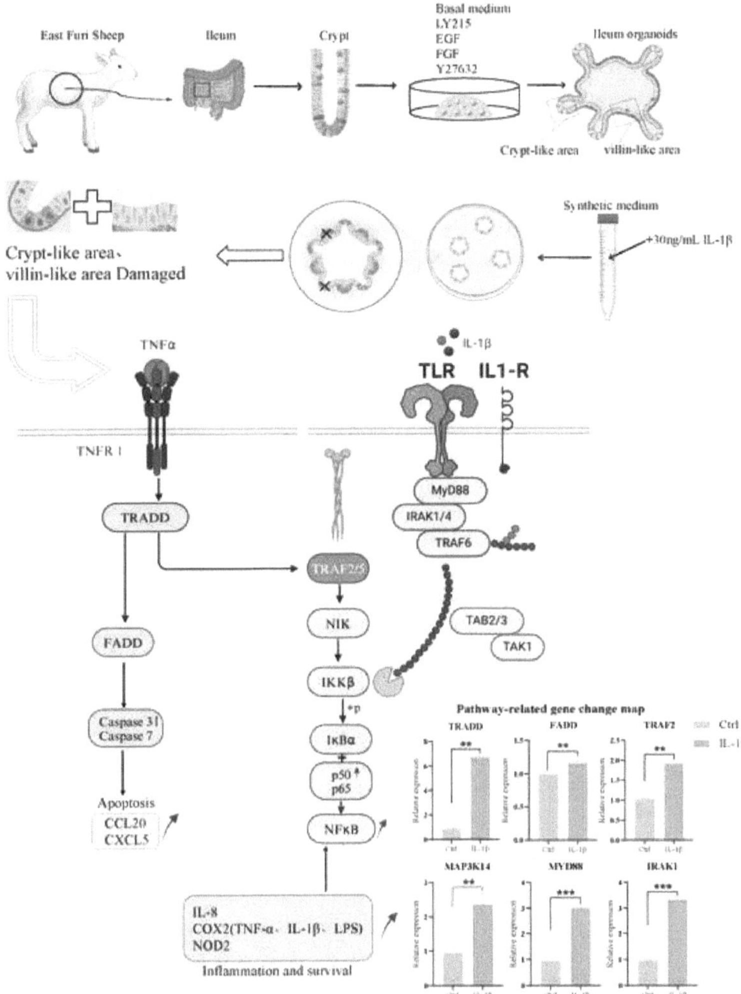

Figure 13 illustrates the comprehensive experimental pattern [225].

Furthermore, although sheep intestinal organoids are capable of mimicking some characteristics of the actual intestinal environment, they ultimately do not completely simulate the intricate physiological and pathological conditions of the entire sheep organism. An example of this limitation is the intricate interactions between the intestine and other bodily organs, as well as the influence of the systemic immune system on the intestine, which may not be accurately portrayed in the organoid model.

Variations may also exist in the response of sheep intestinal organoids to specific stimuli compared to real-time in vivo conditions [226, 227].

Cytokines and Cytokine Targeting in Sepsis: From Humans to Horses

The costs and mortality rates associated with adult and neonatal sepsis in both humans and horses are considerable. From 2004 to 2018, the mortality rates for human adult sepsis were reported to be 111.8 per 1,000,000 population. In contrast, neonatal mortality rates were as high as 3930 per 100,000 births during the period 2009–2018. Among horses, mortality from sepsis ranges from 37 to 79% in adults depending on the cause, and neonatal sepsis is a major reason for referral to specialized centers and mortality in foals [228, 229].

In the field of human medicine, sepsis is described as a critical organ dysfunction resulting from an uncontrolled immune response to infection, often triggered by the release of endotoxins from gram-negative bacteria or exotoxins from gram-positive bacteria into the bloodstream.

The definition of sepsis in equine medicine is a subject of ongoing discussion, due to the challenges in definitively diagnosing an infection even during severe systemic inflammatory response (SIRS). While there is no universally agreed upon definition of sepsis in horses, some research has adapted the SIRS criteria from human medicine to recognize horses with SIRS/sepsis based on abnormalities in body temperature, heart rate, respiratory rate, and white blood cell count.

Although there is some consensus among equine professionals on SIRS criteria, there is still no definitive definition of sepsis and organ dysfunction, in spite of recent studies by Roy et al. to consider SIRS parameters and results in cases of 479 emergency cases of adult horses [230-233].

The importance of the present research is that it showed that horses that meet every four SIRS criteria and have signs of impaired tissue perfusion have the worst survival chances. The results offer significant clinical implications and outcome evidence that support the significance of the abnormal tissue perfusion in the evolution of the severe SIRS, such as sepsis. The use of these findings must be urgent by equine healthcare practitioners and researchers to adopt a unified set of diagnostic criteria of sepsis in equine patients.

In the past, sepsis has been conceptualized as excessive systemic inflamy as a response to the invading pathogens. Recent studies show that this early hyperinflammatory step is followed by a lengthy phase of immune suppression otherwise known as immune paralysis.

Recent academic publications involving both human subjects and animals have devoted more and more attention to the mechanisms of cytokine production and the possible implications of cytokine hyperproduction in the case of sepsis. This increased understanding in the biomedical sphere has triggered the desire to establish new treatment measures to be directed at cytokines, including cytokine removal and immunomodulation methods in the treatment of sepsis.

A literature search in PubMed, August 1, 2019 until August 1, 2024, has found 1,513 studies focusing on the similarities between medical interventions in humans and horses with their common pathologies with regard to sepsis. Up to now, no universally proven treatment has been found, which completely eliminates sepsis.

This leads to the recommendations of the further studies of the roles of cytokines in sepsis and the possible benefits of cytokine modulation methods as the therapeutic solution. The processes that were explained in this analysis may be used as a basis to conduct future research on the issue of cytokine modulation in humans and equines. [234, 235].

Pathophysiology of Sepsis and Cytokines Roles

A wide range of cells, such as immune cells including macrophages, neutrophils, dendritic cells, T lymphocytes and B lymphocytes and non-immune cells, including endothelium, epithelium and fibroblasts, secrete cytokines which are small soluble proteins. The proteins are essential to cellular signalling, as well as because of the activation of the immune system.

Sepsis is characterised by a severe disturbance of cytokines, which leads to adverse outcomes, including disturbed apoptosis, increased reactive oxygen species, and dysregulated signalling in immune cells. The supporting evidence that high plasma levels of cytokines in sepsis are significantly related to disease severity and mortality of the patients is supported by clinical trials and meta-analysis of literature across several species [236- 240].

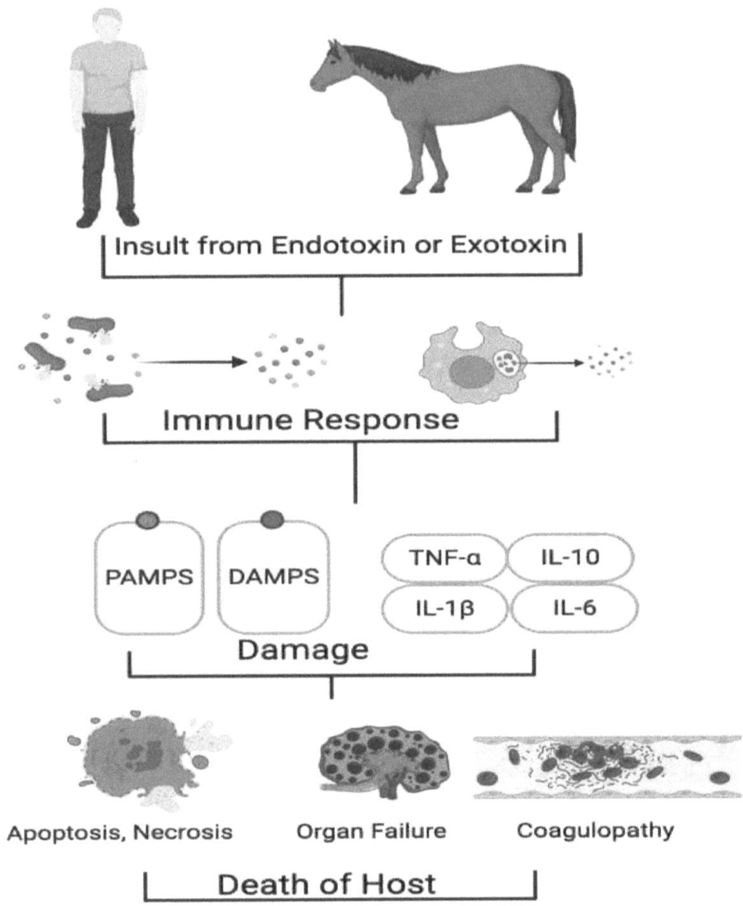

Figure 14shows the similarities in the pathology of humans and horses. [241].

The anti-inflammatory effects of interleukin -6 on T-cell differentiation and inflammatory cytokines release are also reported. The studies by Viva et al. and Molano et al. have found that in the early phase of the disease, high levels of IL-6 in the blood of patients with septic shock are associated with the severity of the disease, dysfunction of the body organs, and mortality. Production of IL 6 in equines is increased during infection especially in sepsis or severe systemic inflammatory response syndrome (SIRS), hence reflecting disease severity and prognosis.

As an example, equines admitting with higher levels of peritoneal IL-6 levels are more prone to organ-related complications, including laminitis, or must be euthanized because of the poor prognosis. In addition, high levels of IL 6 have been observed in the serum of a mare with placentitis and in a horse with equine metabolic syndrome [242-253].

Interleukin-1 beta is a strong initiator of inflammatory response and immune activation and a major mediator of Systemic Inflammatory Response Syndrome (SIRS). This cytokine was produced by activated macrophages and is involved in a number of cellular processes such as proliferation, differentiation, and programmed cell death. Even though IL-1 b might be beneficial in times of stress, its overproduction or continuous overproduction leads to more morbidity and even mortality. A study conducted by Gou et al. established the reposition of CD11c-CD45RBhigh dendritic cells (DCs) and bone-marrow cells (BMCs) under parabiosis mouse models through the action of IL-1b. These results indicate that IL-1B plays a role in sepsis protection by facilitating local BMCs proliferation and differentiation to CD11c-CD45RBhigh DCs in immune and non-immune vessels in sepsis [254-259].

Tumor necrosis factor- alpha has varied effects on various cell and tissues. It increases production of other pro-inflammatory cytokines (IL-1b, IL-6) as well as increases expression of factors that mediate migration of leukocytes to inflamed tissues. Also, TNF -a controls cell death, which facilitates the apoptosis of certain cell types, such as tumor and infected cells.

These discoveries align with the mounting evidence suggesting that TNF-α production during sepsis can lead to vascular damage by promoting abnormal widening and narrowing of blood vessels, which subsequently contributes to organ damage including acute kidney injury in septic horses. Moore et al. also observed that higher levels of TNF-α are linked to unfavorable outcomes in cases of equine colic, though sepsis was not specifically assessed as a complicating factor in those instances [260- 266].

IL-10 is known for its strong anti-inflammatory characteristics. Nevertheless, adult horses subjected to experimentally induced endotoxemia did not show a significant rise in IL-10 gene expression in whole blood when compared to baseline levels at any given time. The contrast in results observed between neonatal and adult horses highlights the current deficiencies in our comprehension of how IL-10 contributes to the progression of endotoxemia and sepsis in equine animals [267-270] .

Cytokine Targeting as a Treatment for Sepsis

Currently, there is a lack of established pharmacological treatment for sepsis, with supportive measures such as antibiotics, cardiovascular support, and corticosteroids being the mainstay of therapy. The uncontrolled inflammatory process that is manifested in sepsis patients highlights the necessity to address cytokines when designing new treatment measures to be applied to the condition.

There are different strategies of cytokine-based therapies, which are anti-inflammatory, anti-endotoxic, and immunomodulatory treatment modalities that have been explored in search of effective sepsis treatments.

The issues related to the possible adverse effects of anti-inflammatory and anti-endotoxic treatment, including renal failures, immunosuppression and epithelial barrier disruption have led to the transition to immune modulation as the major theme of present sepsis-management studies.

In the last five years, the United States National Library of Medicine has registered a significant number of clinical trials with respect to sepsis and cytokines. Currently, there are 293 clinical trials enrolled on cytokine-modulation therapy. Out of those trials, 169 were launched between 1 August 2014 and 1 August 2024, when the data gets filtered concerning the past ten years. The hemoperfusion therapy to remove cytokines is the main concern in 29 of these clinical trials. Using the PubMed database, one was able to find 12,028 publications that highlighted cytokine targeting as a key mechanism of therapy by searching the database with the terms sepsis, cytotokines, and the time period between 1 August 2019 and 1 August 2024.

This database analysis suggests that most of the immunomodulatory therapeutic interventions against sepsis can be divided into three groups:

monoclonal-antibody therapy, cytokine-receptor-blockade, or cytokine-elimination [271].

Monoclonal antibody therapy

In a study that included a model of endotoxemia induced experimentally in miniature horses, the group that was administered with monoclonal antibodies targeting tumor necrosis factor -alpha exhibited a significant decrease in the plasma concentration of TNF -alpha relative to the control group. Moreover miniature horses treated with TNF- 2 monoclonal antibodies scored low on clinical anomalies, reduced heart rates, and elevated white blood cell count compared to those receiving isotype control monoclonal antibodies.

This study was found to have an influence on the production of interleukin-6, lactate and prostacyclin by the administration of the anti-TNF-a monoclonal antibody therapy to the miniature horses that were infused with lipopolysaccharide.

In more recent studies, the efficacy of antiphosphatase of interleukin (anti IL-5 monoclonal antibodies) in adjunctive therapy of horses with insect bite hypersensitivity has been investigated.

Cytokine/cytokine receptor (C5A) targeted monoclonal antibody has demonstrated effectiveness in reducing the need to be hospitalized and to undergo mechanical ventilation in patients with COVID-19. However, it is also important to note that in 2022 the Food and Drug Administration banned the use of many monoclonal antibodies as a means of treating COVID-19 because of adverse reactions issues, which reflects the potentially harmful impact of blocking the normal functioning of the body with regard to dealing with infections [272- 276].

The cytokine antagonists

The cytokine antagonists have the ability to block the cytokine activity by different mechanisms such as direct interaction with the receptors to induce a long lasting immune blockage, regulation of the cytokine production, and binding to the cytokines to block further actions.

IL-6 receptor inhibition has been linked to a decrease in mortality rate and critical care admission of sepsis in the context of human sepsis.

Moreover, CXCR1 receptor has been shown to reduce lung injury, thrombosis and neutrophil extracellular traps production in human and murine sepsis models. Although the therapy of cytokine antagonists in horses is still largely limited to osteoarthritis, with an IL-1 receptor antagonist, the positive results reported in suppressing inflammatory pathways indicate that there is potential to discuss the implementation of cytokine antagonists therapy in the treatment of sepsis.

Though cytokine antagonists usually have been considered as the cheaper substitute to monoclonal antibodies targeting cytokines, it is noteworthy that such therapies may exhibit similar adverse reactions because of the attenuated ability to fight infections [277-280].

Cytokine Removal

Of increasing interest is the elimination of circulating cytokines in septic patients through extracorporeal hemoperfusion therapy, monoclonal antibodies or antagonist drugs to block cytokines or cytokine receptors. This treatment method involves the circulation of anticoagulated blood through a column with a filter medium with the assistance of a peristaltic pump and its reintroduction into the patient.

Hemoperfusion therapy is seen to be a more conservative method of effectively treating cytokines in the context of suspected patients with sepsis than the alternative therapy used in treating patients like monoclonal antibodies and cytokine antagonists that may lead to prolonged immune suppression.

An emerging literature suggests that hemoperfusion can also play a beneficial role in minimizing tissue damage associated with leukocytes by eliminating circulating neutrophil extracellular traps as well as by preventing neutrophil-reactive oxygen species. The systems of hemoperfusion therapy work through three major mechanisms: non-selective bead binding, selective bead binding, or binding to a permeable membrane [281- 283].

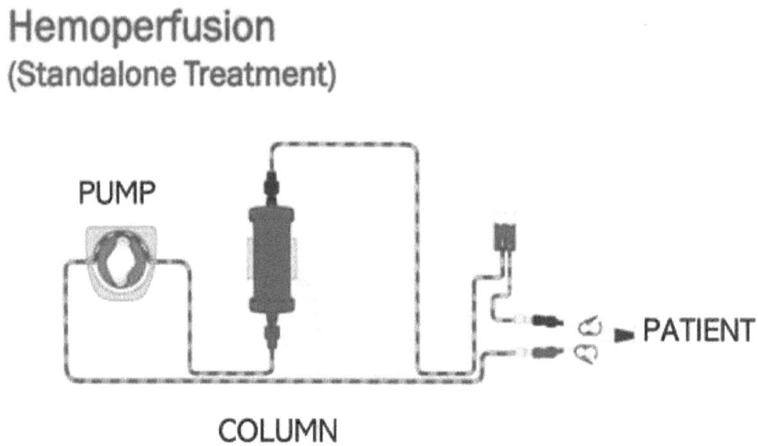

Figure 15 demonstrates the hemoperfusion process whereby blood is removed off the patient, filtered in a given column and later returned to the circulation of the patient.

In the nonselective binding, molecules that have the size between 5 and 60kD are effectively filtered out.

Nonselective devices based on polymer use a concentration-dependent gradient to remove inflammatory cytokines, thus providing a more effective clearance of high plasma concentrations but not full clearance, which may be harmful since the cytokines are vital to immunological functionality.

Those studies have demonstrated that hemoperfusion using a polymer-based column (CytoSorb) has the potential to significantly decrease cytokine levels in patients with inflammation caused by sepsis, eventually leading to a decreased mortality rate and a lower rate of vasoplegic shock in the patients under extracorporeal life support, and to a reduction in the need of mechanical ventilation in patients with COVID-19.

On the contrary, nonselective activated-carbon ones do not work on a gradient-removal principle but on a mesoporous structure to adsorb cytokines.

Even though the activated-carbon filters showed only a limited influence on cytokine levels in clinical trials that were conducted on human subjects, the devices have shown to be effective in eliminating endotoxins in the blood after hemoperfusion.

A polymer- based apparatus (VetResQ) has shown the ability to remove ex vivo cytokines in LPS-stimulated equine blood and is also safe when implanted in adult equine in experiments and clinical trials.

The use of hemoperfusion columns filled with polymyxin B (Toraymyxin) has been linked to a decrease of mortality rates amongst human cases of septic shock.

A more modern line is currently in place with permeable-membrane devices which bind cytokines and endotoxins to remove them by membrane adherence.

These devices provide similar advantages as traditional dialysis such as removal of creatinine and uremic toxins, and current clinical trials assess their overall effectiveness. [**291**,**292**].

Transcutaneous stimulation of the vagal nerve of the ear was done in alert and healthy horses.

A number of factors and mechanisms have been linked to the occurrence of POI, some of which include anesthetic agents, opioids, intravenous fluids, electrolyte imbalances, GI hormones neuropeptides disruption, neural discontinuity, autonomic impairment, and inflammatory cell activation. The pathogenesis of POI has been now recognized to have two phases; firstly, an early neurogenic phase, which directly affects bowel movement following surgery, and secondly, an inflammatory phase, which can last several days. Even though these stages are distinct phases of the POI development, a well known mutual interaction between nervous and immune systems is evident that may possibly lead to a reversal of the ileus.

The abdominal surgery is used as a stimulus where incision, peritoneal breach, and handling of the intestines are considered as some of the stimuli, which activate a sympathetic efferent response, owing to the infliction of pain, and finally causes a reduction of GI motility. This GI motor inhibition is short-term and the normal functioning of the body can be restored, as soon as the painful and pressure sensors stimulation diminishes. The later inflammatory response, in turn, has a more long lasting and devastating effect on intestinal motility [292-294].

Paraphrased text:

The post-operative ileus (POI) has turned into a critical and complicated issue in the clinical care of both veterinary and human patients. Recent studies in specialized veterinary centers in Europe and the United States have found different incidences of POI in horses due to emergency laparotomy with a rate of 0% to 20 %. POI emergence has a significant impact on the hospitalisation period, treatment cost, and future health conditions of individual patients.

Despite its complex etiology, there is currently no standardized approach to managing POI. The existing preventive and treatment protocols in equine medicine, which predominantly involve supportive care such as anti-inflammatory medications, prokinetic agents, antimicrobial drugs, and intravenous fluid administration, often yield unsatisfactory results [294- 300].

Several studies involving human subjects have provided support for the idea that auricular acupuncture can impact vagal tone. Through transcutaneous auricular vagal nerve stimulation (tAVNS), a non-invasive procedure that involves stimulating the auricular branch of the vagus nerve (ABVN), there is a reduction in systemic inflammation. The ABVN has been known to have an effect on intestinal motility for many years and is sometimes referred to as Alderman's nerve, a nod to the traditional practice of Aldermen in the city of London who would encourage guests at ceremonial banquets to place a rosewater-moistened napkin behind their ears, believing it would aid in digestion. [**301- 305**].

Currently, there is a dearth of information pertaining to the utilization of tAVNS in equine subjects, as well as a detailed anatomical comprehension of the auricular branch of the vagus nerve (ABVN) in horses. The aim of this investigation was to assess the feasibility of employing tAVNS in healthy, non-sedated horses, with the ultimate objective of evaluating the influence of tAVNS on the autonomic nervous system. The examination of heart rate variability (HRV) served as a method to gauge vagus nerve stimulation both before, during, and after the implementation of tAVNS techniques.

The experiment was separated into three different stages, namely: the selection of mares able to endure the manipulation of their ears; the familiarization of those mares with the ear manipulation needed to administer tAVNS; and the stimulation of tAVNS in the selected mares. The stimulation was 90 minutes with continuous heart -rate variability being recorded.

During the first stage, mares were presented with an environment of the stable that they were familiar with where they could have water and grass hay. Gentleness was exercised by the handlers to determine the tolerance of each mare to the position of adhesive electrode needed to stimulate transcutaneous auricular vagus nerves (tAVNS). Mares showing signs of intolerance, e.g. leaping, shaking head, pacing, not wanting to be handled, etc., were immediately left out of the study. Those mares that did not react adversely then went through the subsequent stage whereby the electrodes were placed on the outside and inside of the right pinna using the adhesive patches used.

During the process, mares were closely observed by the handlers in case they felt uncomfortable. In case of distress, the machine was turned off as quickly as possible, the patches were taken off and the mare was discontinued in the research. The mares that were quiet and compliant during the adaptation phase only proceeded to the final phase, where they were kept in the stable with the TENS device as passive [306].

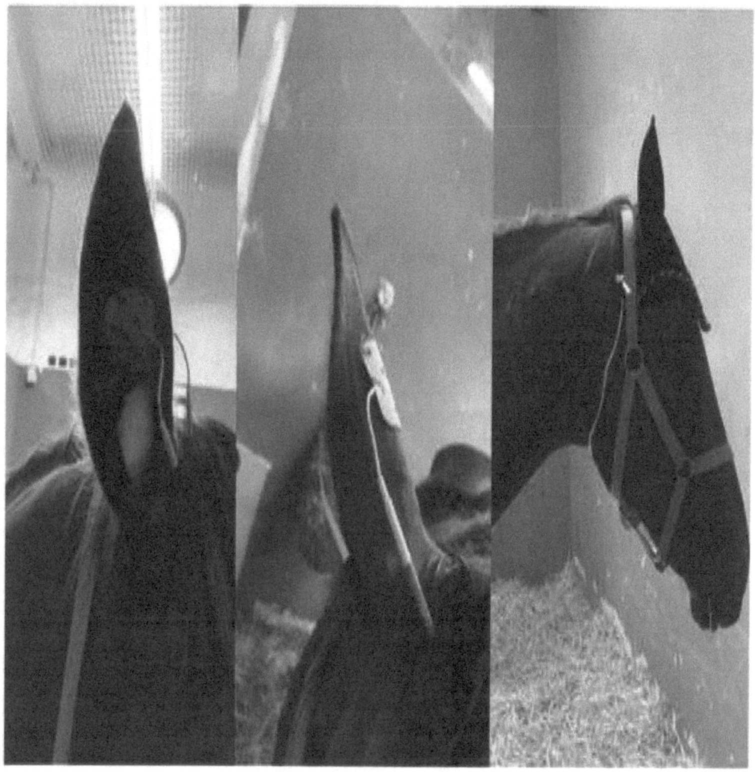

Figure 16 shows how two adhesive electrodes have been applied to the external and internal parts of the right pinna.

This application was preceded by using cotton balls in order to pad the ears, then an ear bonnet was put over the head.

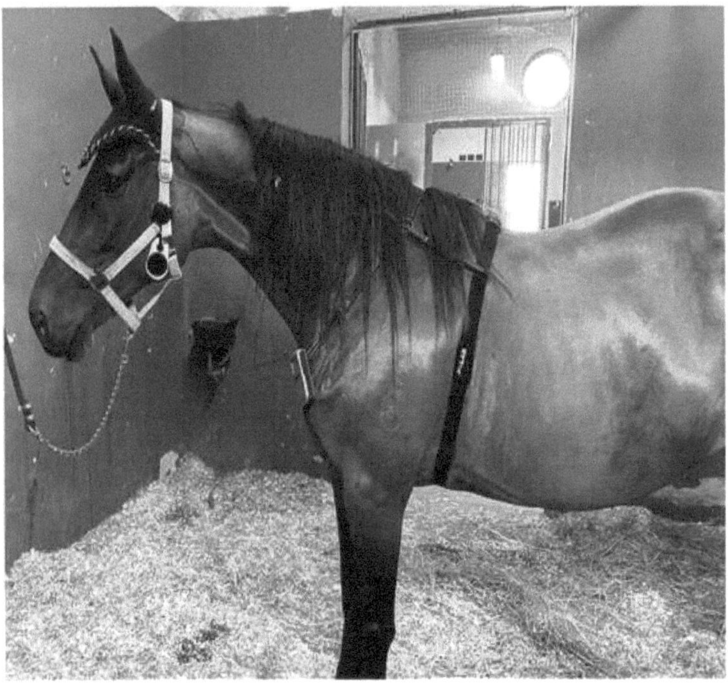

Figure 17 illustrates how the TENS device should be placed on a cervical collar and the polar belt is placed on the thoracic area behind the elbow, and ultrasound gel is applied to the electrodes.

During the whole ninety minutes, an operator monitored the behavior of the mares outside of the stable, ready to take any action in case any signs of discomfort, including vocalizing, circling, and jumping, were exhibited by the subjects. The mares were allowed to roam freely in the stall and water was made available to them but no food was given.

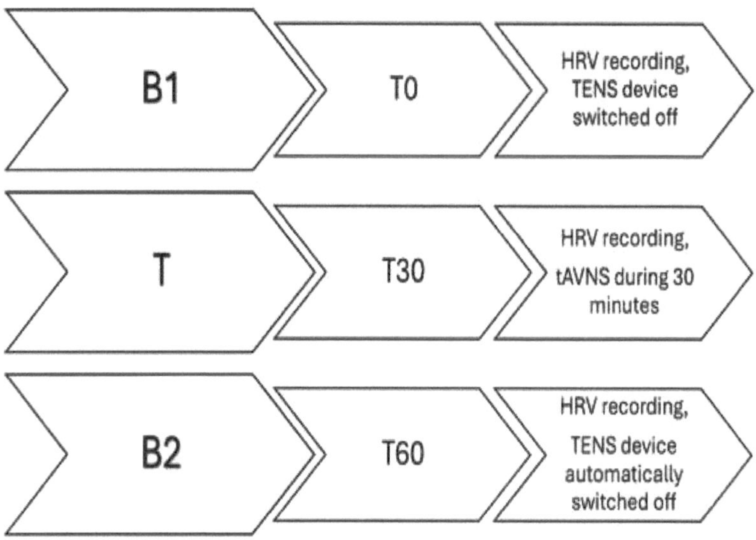

Figure 18 depicts a visual breakdown of the three stages comprising the third phase of the study.

The sympathetic nervous system index (SNSi) was determined by evaluating the average heart rate, STi, and non-linear analysis of the length of Poincaré plot distribution. Conversely, the parasympathetic nervous system index (PNSi) was determined by assessing mean interbeat intervals, RMSSD through time-domain analysis, and the width of Poincaré plot distribution [**407- 309**].

A total of 22 out of 44 mares were able to tolerate the manipulation of their ears and advance to the second phase of the study. However, among these 22 mares, only 10 were able to progress to the third phase as 12 mares did not respond well to the tAVNS treatment. Additionally, three mares had to be excluded during HRV recordings due to displaying signs of discomfort and an elevated heart rate of over 80 bpm.

The tolerance of the female horses involved in the research towards the transcutaneous electrical nerve stimulation (TENS) device was examined, and its impact on the autonomic nervous system was assessed by analyzing heart rate variability (HRV). Many horses display sensitivity when it comes to their ears, which can present challenges in handling them. Reasons for ear sensitivity can vary, ranging from physical to behavioral issues, although the investigation of the specific causes was not within the scope of this study.

The remaining 37 out of 44 mares were excluded due to displaying discomfort during one of the three stages. As mental stress is known to be linked to a decrease in parasympathetic tone, it was deemed unfair to continue with the study protocol as it could compromise the well-being of the horses and go against the research objectives. To validate the poor tolerance of awake horses of this species to tAVNS, a broader sample of horses from varied breeds and sexes should be tested [310]

Therefore, it is speculated that electrical stimulation at any point on the ear could activate vagal afferent fibers. In the absence of specific anatomical guidance, it was believed that any area of the ear could potentially stimulate the vagus nerve, and the external and internal surfaces of the pinna were deemed suitable for the application of the adhesive patches. [301, 302, 306].

The findings suggest that there was greater vagal stimulation and significant sympathetic withdrawal in B2, indicated by variations in PNSi and SNSi. The indices are based on the heart rate and other heart-rate-variability parameters, which make them susceptible to bias during interpretation by an analyst.

The separation of two subgroups with autonomic reactions that were different was done through the examination of each equine subject results.

This is despite the fact that a behavioral variability was not observed, yet, the Group A, in comparison to the Control, showed an increase in heart rate and a decrease in time-domain HRV parameters throughout the intervention, suggesting reduced parasympathetic with increased sympathetic activity, which is the opposite of what should have occurred to the tAVNS.

These results should therefore be used with caution when inferences are made on the autonomic function.

The study established that tAVNS enhanced vagal tone only in four out of seven mares.

The side effects reported in human subjects that are linked with the tAVNS include cutaneous irritation, pruritus, tinnitus, cephalalgia, and nasopharyngitis.

Even though no cases of cutaneous irritation or pruritus in mares undergoing tAVNS was noted in this study, tinnitus or cephalalgia may have occurred in a subset of the mares that may explain the effects of increasing heart rate and reducing HRV in Group A during therapy.

It is reasonable to believe that, regardless of being provoked by vagal nerve stimulation, the electromechanical vibration used by the TENS device might have caused discomfort in such mares, even though no behavioral changes were observed.

Further studies ought to consider using a reduced pulse to determine the stimulation threshold needed to activate the vagal stimulation and avoid the side effects [314].

Simultaneously, numerous investigations of the effect of TENS on the human autonomic nervous system have produced conflicting results, which can be primarily explained by changes in the frequency, intensity, and point of application of stimulation.

In its turn, these discrepancies may trigger vagal afferents to varying degrees.

The vagus nerve is a combination of A, B, and C fiber of which unmyelinated C fibers make up the maximum of 70-80% of the total fibers, requiring intensities of stimulation and lower frequencies to activate.

Direct stimulation of C fibers usually causes bradycardia, but A fibers are the major stimulus of TENS, which inhibits the transmission of nociceptive by stimulating C fibers.

The apparent inefficacy of tAVNS in some patients may be explained by interindividual variation in the amount of myelinated A axons in the venauralgural nerve in the ear.

The same principle could be applied to the horses, and therefore the difference in the rate of variability of the heart rate (HRV) of the groups A and B can be explained. Without certain anatomical researches on this species, transcutaneous activation of the vagus nerve by the use of transcutaneous auricular vagus nerve stimulation (tAVNS) in horses might not be as effective as in humans [315320].

More so, the discovery of vagus nerve stimulation being able to dampen the inflammatory response of a sepsis model has additionally indicated that a cholinergic anti-inflammatory pathway might exist. The net result of these two functions of the vagus nerve to stimulate muscular locomotion and to suppress the inflammatory response presents a desirable approach to the control of intestinal motility and immune reaction after abdominal surgery in human and equine patients. Since there are no findings to prove the use of tAVNS in awake horses, whose auditory system is very sensitive, its efficacy can be explored in the scenario of general anaesthesia of acute cases of the gastrointestinal tract, or during the immediate post-surgical period when the residual effects of the anaesthesia may impair auditory-system sensitivity [321323].

There are a number of limitations in this study. To start with, the third phase dealt with a limited sample of animals, thus, restricting the statistical strength of the results and requiring other results to be confirmed in a larger population. Secondly, the observations of animal behaviour were conducted solely by the involved veterinarians, and no further recordings and objective assessment were carried out. Although we could see a significant difference in behaviour of the horses, which tolerated ear touch and electrical stimulation compared to those, which did not, it could be possible that minor differences were ignored, which may explain the differences in HRV between group A and B. Besides, the researchers did not investigate other potential outcomes of vagal stimulation, which includes intestinal motility and fecal production. Measurement of fecal product would have involved prolonged housing of mares which was not feasible because of institutional limitations. In addition, the abdominal auscultation in tAVNS was discouraged to eliminate the effects of human relationships with HRV recordings. [307]

Porcine Large Animal Model of Muscular Insufficiency

The significant damage or inflammation of skeletal muscles may result in chronic muscle weakness and great loss of the quality of life. Stress urinary incontinence (SUI) is one of the clear cut cases of chronic conditions, which occur as a result of muscular weakness, in addition to other disorders. SUI as a disabling condition is found in over 15% of the elderly in our societies and is linked to emotional distress and possible social isolation.

In addition, SUI poses a problem to both medical practitioners and healthcare systems. In females, antecedent factors including pregnancy, childbirth and menopause lead to SUI, as opposed to men where antecedents are often the result of prostate surgery. SUI also may affect both sexes due to the lower pelvic area injury or chronic inflammation of urogenital organs, neurological conditions, aging, and cognitive impairment. The SUI therapy aims at strengthening the muscles affected or improving the functionality of the affected muscles through the various modalities. Lower pelvic floor and electrophysiological stimulation therapy with the use of physical exercises have proven to be promising in improving muscle strength and possibly solving SUI in its mild forms.

Behavioral therapy skills and pharmacologic treatments are some of the non-surgical methods used to treat SUI. In case these modalities do not prove beneficial in meeting the needs of the patient, surgery might be justified. The interventions vary significantly between female and male patients and include injection of bulking agents, tailor-made tapes or slings and artificial sphincters. However, such interventions have intrinsic risks of peri-operative and long-term outcomes, and they do not correct etiologies of SUI. One of the central aspects of the processes of SUI development is a functional tissue loss of muscles or insufficient muscle contraction in the Urethral closure complex, so the study of the minimally invasive cell-based process of muscle regeneration becomes an important subject. Myoblasts are considered to be promising materials in the healing of the lacking urethral sphincter complex [328-337].

Myoblasts cultured in an optimal environment were pretransplanted into a porcine model with sphincter muscle insufficiency before it was observed that the sphincter was regenerating. [338- 340].

Porcine muscle-derived cell populations Isolation and in vitro culture

Young boars were chosen since they have a greater concentration of these cells within the musculature as compared to old pigs. The tissue samples have been removed under strict aseptic conditions, stored in transport media and put in sterile containers, transported to the lab within an hour in wet ice [339, 340] (Figure 21).

The microscopic observations of the cells were done on a basis of their phenotypic features. The determination of the duplication rate (DR) was done by washing, detaching the cells with trypsin -EDTA, suspended the cells in media, counting them with the trypan blue exclusion in a hematocytometer, and seeded them at a density of 2-105 cells/flask.

Differentiation process and development of syncytia or long fiber-like cells were studied using a microscope [339, 340].

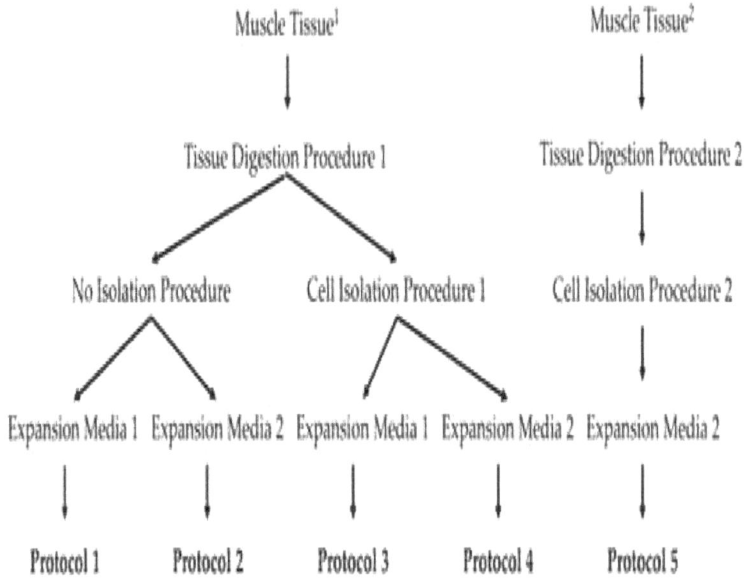

Figure 19 is a diagram that shows how five protocols were implemented. [340].

Assessment of Gene Expression at the Transcript Level

To ready up to RNA extraction, the growth medium used in the process of cell expansion was washed away and the myoblasts stuck to the surface washed twice with phosphate-buffered saline (PBS). Subsequently, the quantitative real-time polymerase chain reaction (qPCR) was carried out on the cDNA sample utilizing gene-specific oligonucleotides, following a procedure outlined in a recent publication.

The housekeeping genes swine glyceraldehyde phosphate dehydrogenase (GAPDH) and β2-microglobulin (b2MG) were employed as internal controls in each run to standardize the expression levels of the target genes. The efficiency-corrected advanced relative quantification program of the LightCycler 480 II, as per the manufacturer's instructions, was utilized for this purpose [341,**342**].

Detection of protein using immunofluorescence techniques

Myoblasts were cultured on chamber slides until they achieved the desired level of confluence. Upon removal of the medium, the cells were rinsed twice with cold PBS, fixed with 4% paraformaldehyde, and permeabilized with 0.1% Triton X-100 at room temperature.

To reduce nonspecific antibody binding, the samples were preincubated with a blocking solution containing 5% dry milk powder in 0.1% Tween-20 in PBS. After removing the blocking solution, the primary anti-desmin antibody was applied at a concentration of 1:200 in 0.1% BSA in PBS and incubated in black humidified chambers at 37°C for 90 minutes.

Any unbound primary antibodies were removed by aspiration, and the samples were then washed three times with T-PBS. The detection antibody (FITC-F(ab')2-dk-anti-rbt IgG (H+L), 1:200) was subsequently added to the samples and incubated in black humidified chambers at 37°C for 45 minutes. Control samples were also prepared without primary antibodies.

Flow Cytometry

The myoblasts were dislodged using a gentle proteolysis technique involving Accutase from SigmaAldrich, St. Louis, MO, USA, with a suspension of 5 × 105 cells being prepared in PFEA sample buffer and transferred to microtubes for sedimentation.

To prevent non-specific antibody binding, the cells were first incubated with pre-immune serum (Gamunex, diluted 1:20 in PBS; 20 minutes, 0 °C; Grifols SA, Barcelona, Spain), followed by washing and subsequent incubation at 0 °C for 20 minutes with a cross-reactive PE-labeled antibody directed against human CD56 (NCAM, diluted 1:10 in PFEA; BioLegend, San Diego, CA, USA).

The size and granularity of the cells were evaluated using flow cytometry, specifically assessing forward scatter (FSC-A) and side scatter (SSC-A) on an LSRII instrument from BD Bioscience in Franklin Lakes, NJ, USA in order to select viable cells. Flow cytometry was then employed to quantify the intensity of antibody staining. Cells without antibody staining, in addition to FC compensation particles from BD Bioscience, were used for gating purposes.

The acquired data was analyzed using FACS-Diva software (version 6.1.3) and FlowJo software (version 10.10), both from BD Bioscience. The FCS and SSC scatters were visualized in 2D dot plots, while the median fluorescence intensity (MFI) of stained cells was presented in histograms with a thin black line, contrasting with the background fluorescence of unstained cells displayed in shaded histograms. [348, 349].

Efficacy of Myoblast Treatment in a Preclinical Animal Trial

For a limited preclinical study on feasibility, one additional male pig and five female landrace pigs were carefully chosen. The myoblasts required for cell therapy were derived from the male pig following the standard protocol outlined in Protocol 4 (Figure 21). The female landrace pigs underwent induction of urethral sphincter muscle deficiency through transurethral electrocautery and balloon dilatation.

Verification of sphincter deficiency was done by measuring the urethral closure pressure immediately post surgery using urodynamics (Aquarius TT, Laborie), and normalization was achieved to 100% of the initial closure pressure levels established before surgery for each female pig.

The myoblasts (a total of $1^{-}\ 10^{6}$ myoblasts with two sub-aliquots of 250 micro-liter) were injected into the damaged urethralsphincter muscle, being guided by the cystoscope using a Williams needle (Boston Scientific).

The use of homologous cells established using a male littermate was an effective way of avoiding rejection caused by female littermate recipients when injected with cells, and immunosuppression is used to eliminate rejection which could introduce bias in the results, especially in small-scale researches.

The existence of the Y chromosome in male cells could since then be identified, should it be considered necessary, through such methods as in situ hybridization [350].

Expansion and Structure of Porcine Muscle Cells

The morphologies of the cells represented a variety (Figure 22). Those cells that were generated with Prot.1 and Prot.3 had wider somata, and were more granular (Figure 22A,C).

Many cells produced using these methods appeared flattened, enlarged, and elongated (Figure 22E). This could resemble characteristics of replicative senescence. Myoblasts cultured using Prot.2, Prot.4, and Prot.5 appeared slender and devoid of prominent granularity (Figure 22 B,D,F).).

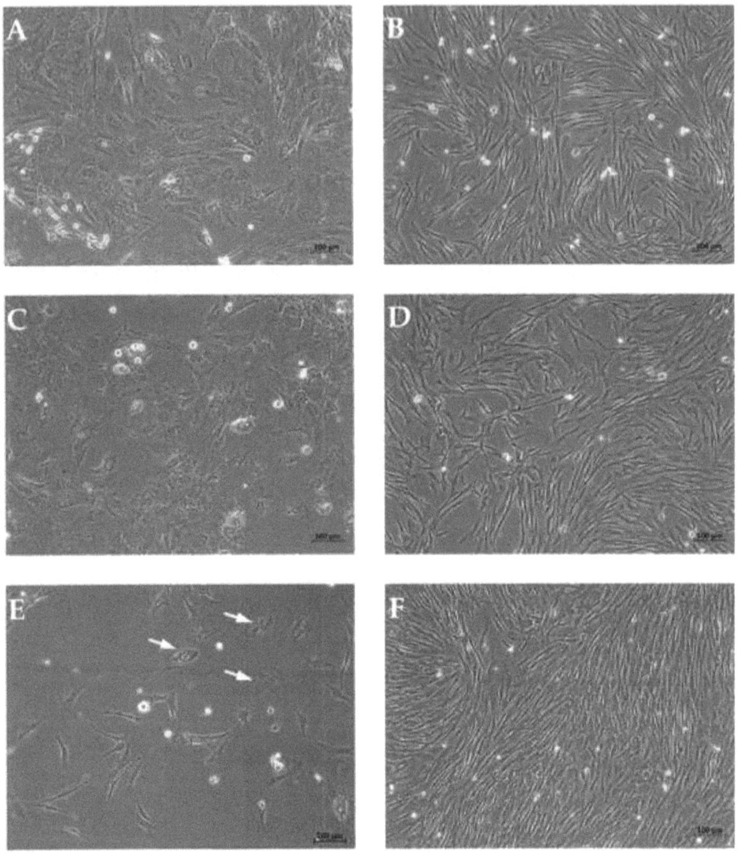

Figure (20): Morphological comparison of myoblasts expanded using various protocols

Expression of genes encoding proteins that are specific markers for muscle formation

Numerous key genes have been identified as being essential in the process of myogenesis. The examination of gene expression, particularly of Pax7 for proliferating myoblasts, and various myogenic regulatory factors such as MyoD1, Myf5, MyoG, Myf6 (MRF4), along with levels of Desmin intermediate filament in muscle, was conducted using RT-qPCR on myoblasts expanded utilizing five distinct protocols. Results indicated that myoblasts produced through Prot.4 demonstrated the highest expression levels of all myogenic markers, followed by those generated through Prot.2 and Prot.5. In contrast, myoblasts generated using Prot.1 and Prot.3 exhibited notably lower levels of marker gene expression [352, 353].

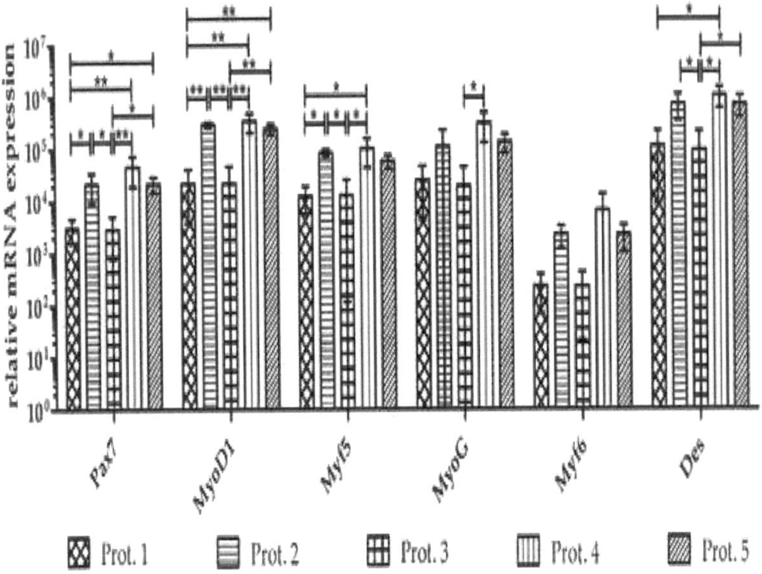

Figure 21 illustrates the transcript expression of myogenic marker genes in myoblasts.

Determination of CD56 by means of Flow Cytometry

Our study revolved around examining the presence of CD56 on porcine myoblasts using flow cytometry in three separate examinations.

The percentage of myoblasts that were found to express CD56 was significantly higher in cells that were grown in D-media than in those that were grown in M-media. Also the average fluorescence intensity (MFI) of myoblasts grown in K-media was lesser than in D-media with maximal levels of expressing being seen in Prot.4 cells.

This suggests that cell propagation in the D-media without horse serum enabled high level of CD56 expression in swine myoblasts [354-356].

Porcine myoblasts Desmin expression

The immunofluorescence showed that all batches of myoblasts prepared in the donors contained desmin (Figure 22 A). Due to the fact that it is impossible to determine the exact value of a particular protein using the intensity of immunofluorescence only, DAPI was used to stain the nuclei in order to be able to distinguish between desmin-positive and desmin-negative myoblasts (Figure 22 B).

The proportions of desmin-positive cells in the myoblast populations obtained through protocols 2 (48.9 ; 3), 4 (49.1 , 3), and 5 (38.7) were significantly greater than those of the ones obtained through protocols 1 (8.2) and 3 (7.4) (Figure 23 B). This observation indicates that culturing of porcine muscle originated cells in D-media is more effective in generating myoblast enriched cultures compared to cultures grown in M-media [357, 358].

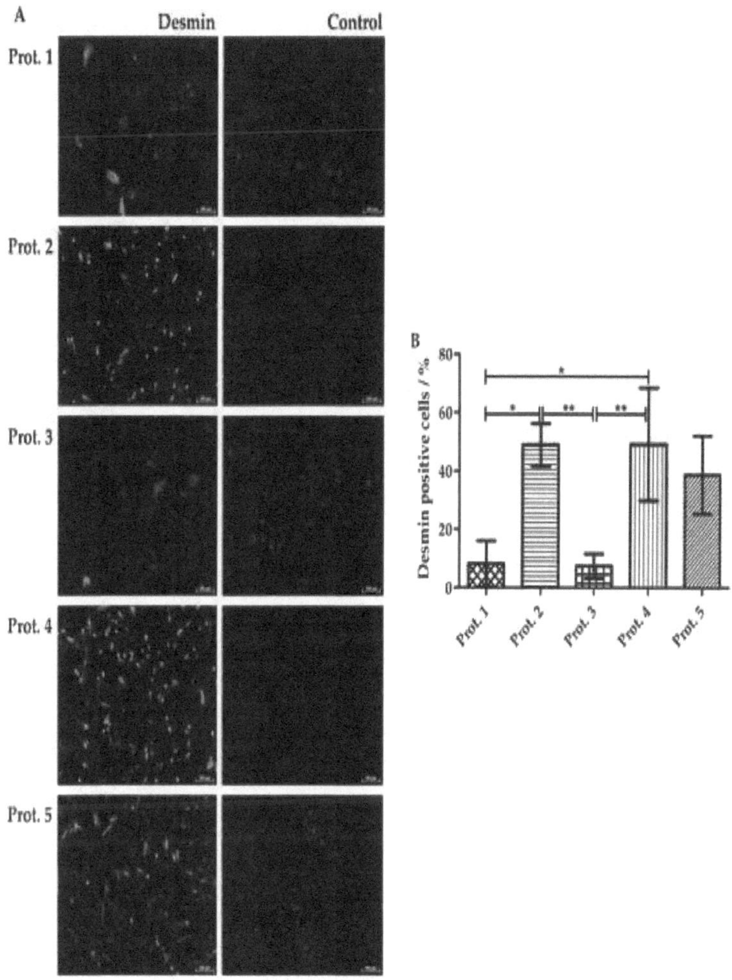

Figure (22): The intracellular desmin was detected by the use of immunofluorescence.

Myogenesis Production of Myotubes through cell differentiation

Myoblasts obtained of cells of three separate donor animals were induced to differentiate into myotubes and proliferate in line with Protocols1 to Protocols5. The myoblasts were then differentiated as per the procedure.

Per Protocols 2, 4 and 5 which led to the expansion of myoblasts, long myotubes expressing desmin were obtained, and at Protocols 1 and 3 which led to the expansion of myoblasts, shorter or non-elongated myotubes were obtained.

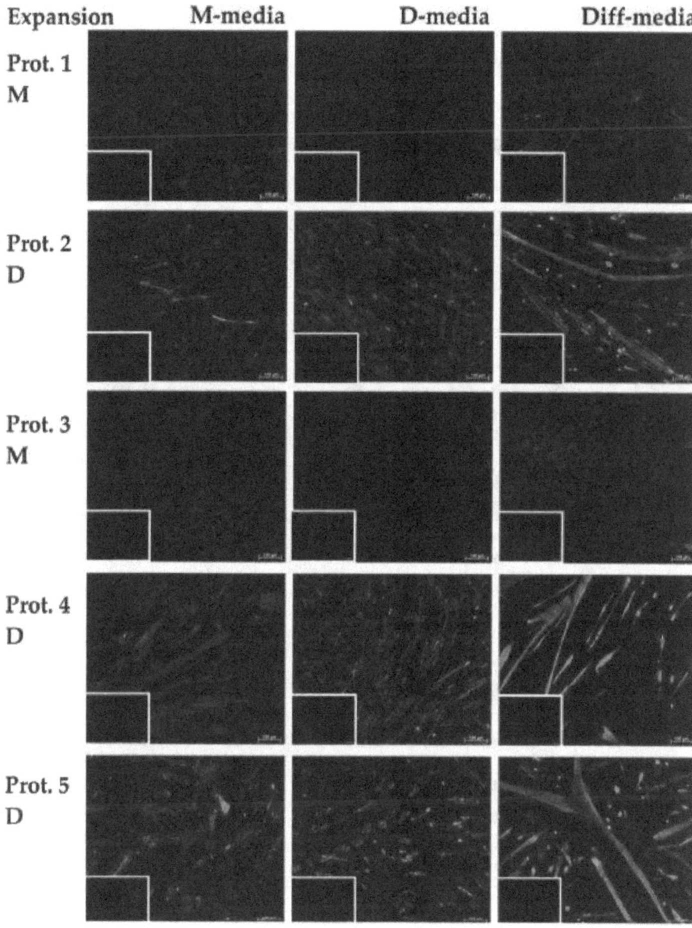

Figure 23 illustrates the process of terminal differentiation of myoblasts.

At the outset, a significant portion of myoblasts grown in M-media using Protocols 1 and 3 exhibited a lack of viability upon transition to D-media. Subsequent DAPI staining revealed a limited presence of viable cells and intact nuclei following the change in media.

Nevertheless, these cells managed to endure the shift to differentiation media, albeit without effective formation of myotubes as shown in Figure 26.

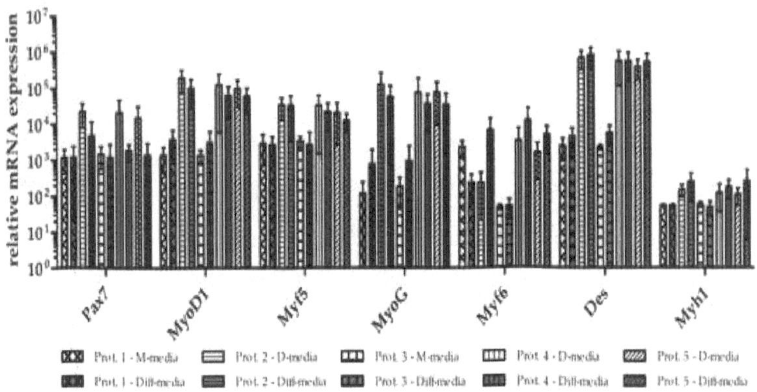

Figure (24): Analysis of marker gene expression in myotubes was conducted through RT-qPCR [359, 360].

Using myoblast therapy to treat a weakened sphincter muscle in an animal model of incontinence

Urinary incontinence was artificially induced in five female pigs through surgical techniques involving transurethral electrocautery and balloon dilatation. The deficiency in the sphincter was then rectified by injecting 1 × 106 myoblasts from the M. semitendinosus muscle of a male littermate using Prot.4 directly into the damaged urethrae.

It was observed that spontaneous recovery from the induced urethral muscle deficiency reached 67.03% ± 14.00% ($p < 0.05$) without myoblast injection. However, utilizing Prot.4 myoblast injection led to a more significant functional regeneration, especially when compared to the urethral wall pressure post-sphincter injury induction.

Further observations revealed that sphincter regeneration facilitated by myoblast injection showed improvement compared to mock-treated controls, although the difference did not reach statistical significance when compared to spontaneous recovery.

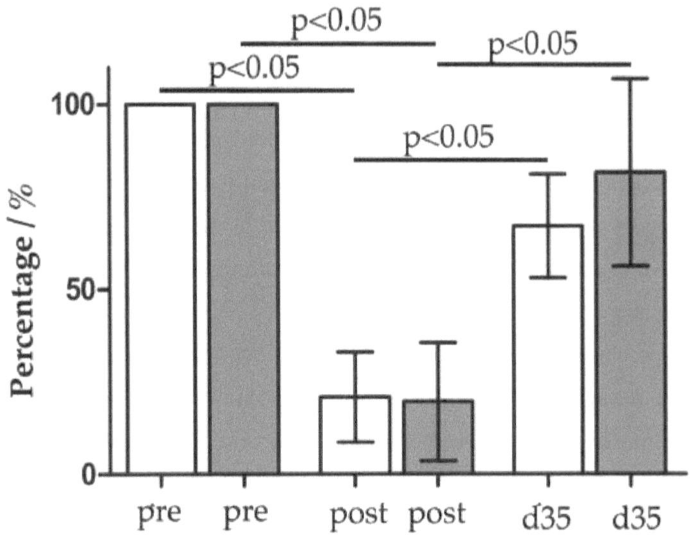

Figure (25) depicts the process of restoring the deficient urethral sphincter muscle through the injection of myoblasts.

The achievements of preclinical animal studies have paved the way for clinical feasibility studies focused on cell therapy for stress urinary incontinence (SUI) using a patient's own cells. Despite initial optimism in the past, cell therapy for SUI has not yet become a standard practice in clinical settings.

Moreover, striated muscle cells, which derive out of the outer rhabdosphincter, reinforce the contractile complex. As a result, stromal cells obtained using adipose tissue or skeletal myoblast as their sources have been utilized [361365].

The production of regenerative-competent human mesenchymal stromal cells using different sources such as bone marrow, adipose tissue and skeletal myoblasts derived out of M. soleus under optimal medical conditions are the leading edge of the technology.

Regrettably, little is known about the production procedures or cell types that have been employed in animal models of stress urinary incontinence (SUI), which is why one cannot interpret outcomes of treatment properly. Although there are some preclinical investigations on myoblasts before the application to SUI models, the lack of in-depth information on the quality indicators of porcine muscle cells used in regenerative therapy research is still significant [366–368–370].

During our early studies we analyzed the phenotype of myoblasts isolated out of the different skeletal muscles in the adult animals and found that there is inefficient expression of the markers in cells obtained out of adult pigs. [371].

It is necessary that future researches are conducted to establish whether senescence in myoblasts of pigs can be ascribed to the composition of M-media. On the other hand, D-media is a mixture of F10 medium that is supplemented with 15 per cent FBS, FGF, and antibiotics, leading to increase in cell proliferation and strong expression of markers of muscle cells [372-374].

The observed death after the change in M-media to D-media, shows that although M-media assists in the growth of the cells, it does not provide the protective effect against cell death. The reduced viability in changing media can be attributed to the lack of some factors of survival. The invasion of cells in tissue may lead to stress although, the increase in the viability was coupled with down regulation of the expression of CD56, which is a gene associated with muscle differentiation and stress resistance. The ability of cells to survive after implantation death is a key factor to success of cell-based therapies which is why the expression of CD56 as a quality parameter should be used when analyzing future myoblast treatment [375- 378].

Comparing the myoblasts of three different boars, we found that there was a difference in the expression of the marker genes, suggesting the possibility of interindividual differences in domestic pigs that could have influence on the cellular characteristics. Such disparities might lead to inconsistent data of clinical cell therapies and to further quality control measures including epigenetic analyses and the choice of regeneration-competent cells e.g. CD56-positive myoblasts to enhance the treatment outcome. Nevertheless, the search of appropriate markers to enrich human myoblasts should be conducted with additional research [379].

In future studies; there is an urgent need to include greater animal groupings and dose response curves. Also, the cells used in this study were of all derived cells of M. semitendinosus muscle. The process of extracting cells in this large muscle is technically easy hence having an obvious advantage.

After successful cloning, these porcine myoblasts can possibly be used in cellular-therapy studies on larger animal models with muscle loss needs, e.g. anal muscle dysfunction related to fecal incontinence and striated-muscle impairments related to accidents, injuries or surgical procedures (including tumor excisions), and, possibly, in myoblast-therapy studies of cardiac events with suitable modifications.

Human activities have contributed towards a significant increase in emissions of different trace elements in the environment since then the Industrial Revolution began

These components have become common throughout the ecosystems especially raising alarm in the scientific world on their abundance in oceans.

These factors are in two broad categories, including essential and non-essential [380-383]. Conversely, non-essential traces are mostly considered harmless at certain levels below certain levels. However, when these limits are crossed, they make them toxic to an extent of hindering necessary physiological processes. Examples of such elements are chromium, silicon and nickel [384].

The marine mammals are at the top of the marine food webs and tend to be useful in bioindicating the presence of ecological contaminants due to their long lifespan and ecological importance. The bottlenose dolphin, due to its wide range and habitat loyalty, its recorded lifecycle and the ability to store metals is of particular interest as an environmental watchdog species. Conversely, the striped dolphin and Risso dolphin which are the two species under this research are pelagic animals and tend to be found in deeper waters and can also amass high levels of the trace elements due to their position as the top predators. [385-408].

The study of the critical levels of trace elements in the tissues of those dolphin species has been conducted only two times, which has necessitated the importance of collecting the entire data on a variety of trace elements.

To define nutritional and toxicological reference values, to make regional comparisons, and to match contaminant levels with mortality occurrences, it is necessary to determine baseline concentrations of trace elements in cetacean tissues. [409 -411].

The aim of the study was to determine the levels of the two important trace elements which are copper (Cu) and zinc (Zn) in various tissues of dolphins stranded in the Croatian Adriatic coast in the period 1995 to 2013. These substances were chosen because of their critical importance in biological mechanisms, as well as, possible negative outcomes in terms of high concentrations. In addition, the research also tried to make a comparison of these results with the available information on cetaceans across the globe. [412].

Within the given period of time, 190 stranded dead dolphins were studied in the Croatian Adriatic coast. These individuals included 159 bottlenose dolphins (Tursiops truncatus), 25 striped dolphins (Stenella coeruleoalba) and 6 Risso dolphins (Grampus griseus) (Figure 29).

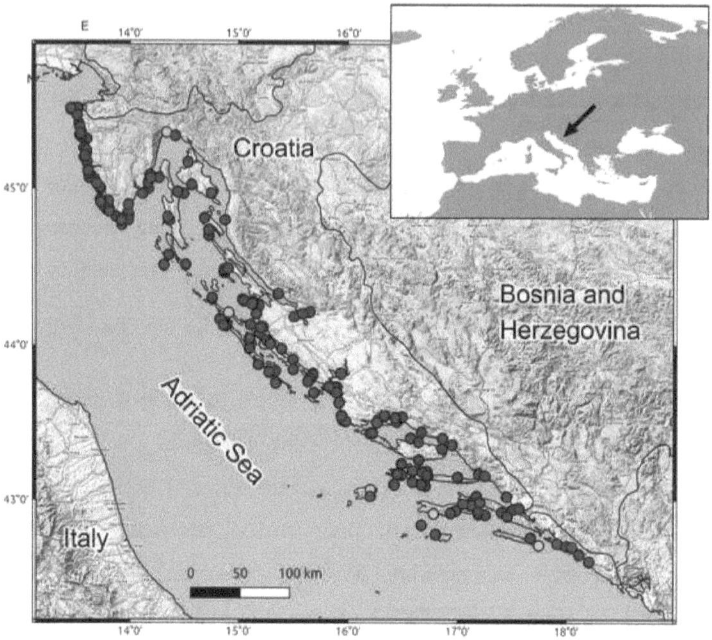

Figure 26 represents the geographical distribution.

In the process of the postmortem examination, a complex of biological and morphometric data were documented including species, sex, body weight, overall body length and other standardized external dimensions. [111 -111[

The copper concentrations in the tissue samples of three species of dolphins were studied

In the assessment of copper levels in bottlenose dolphins based on age and sex, the same level was usually seen within groups with the exception of liver and lung tissues.

Males of adult dolphins showed higher levels of copper concentrations in the liver than females, 17.6-mg/kg and 13.3-mg/kg, respectively.

On the other hand, the juvenile females had higher copper content in liver than juvenile males with 24.9mg/kg and 21.3mg/kg respectively. Also, in lung tissue, juvenile males were found to be higher than juvenile females, 5.32 mg /kg and 2.97 mg /kg, respectively.

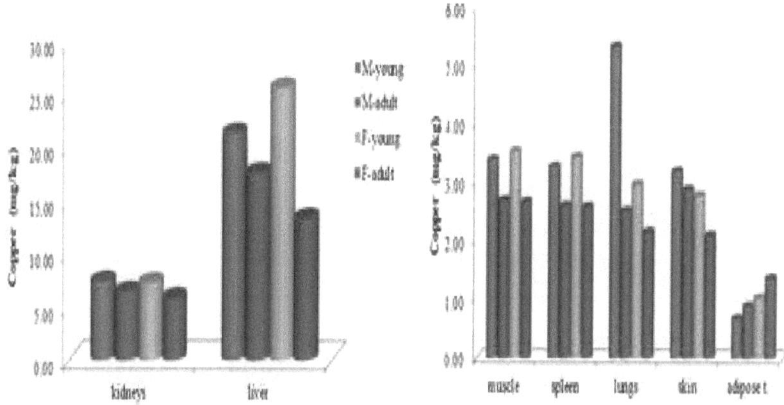

Figure 27 shows the average copper levels in the tissues of bottle nose dolphins, which are grouped on the basis of sex and age.

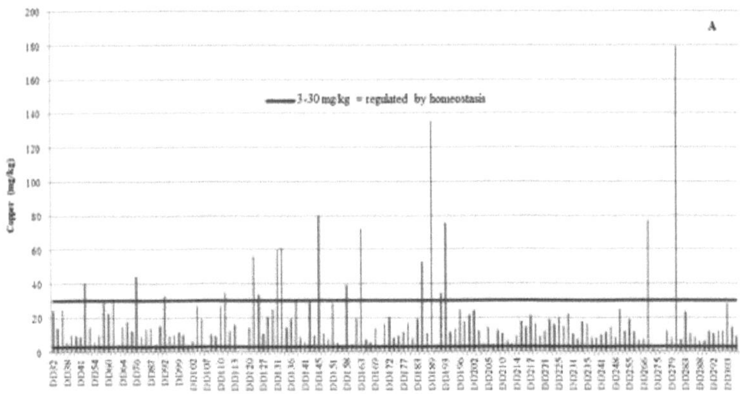

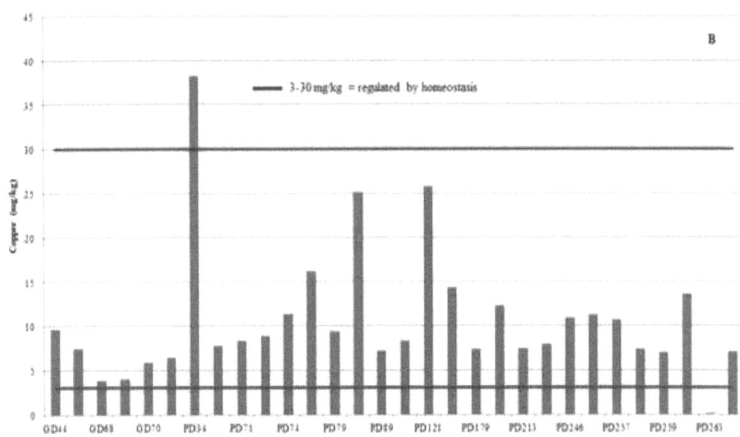

Figure 28 shows the levels of copper (Cu) in the livers of bottlenose dolphins, striped dolphins and Risso dolphins compared to the set critical concentration levels.

Zinc Levels in the Tissues of Three Dolphin Species

The levels of zinc in the different tissues of the three dolphin species had predictable pattern: skin liver kidney other organs.

The interconnection between the system and the environment results in the creation of this cycle.<|human|>The interaction of system and environment leads to the formation of this cycle. (Figure 32)

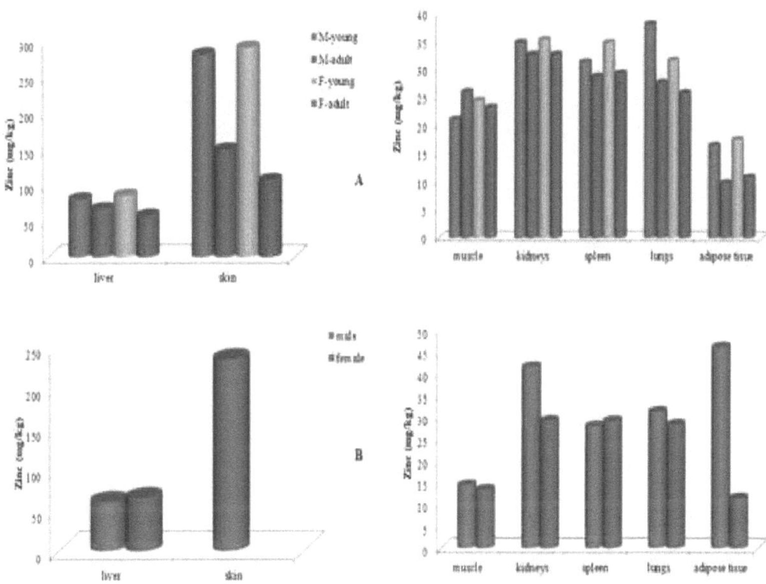

Figure 29 shows the average zinc (Zn) levels in the tissues of bottlenose dolphins.

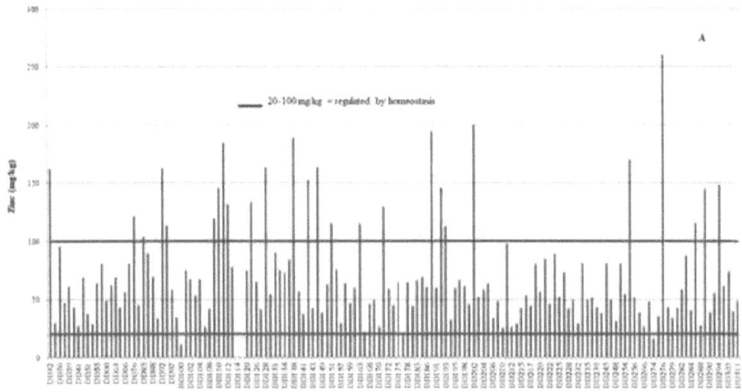

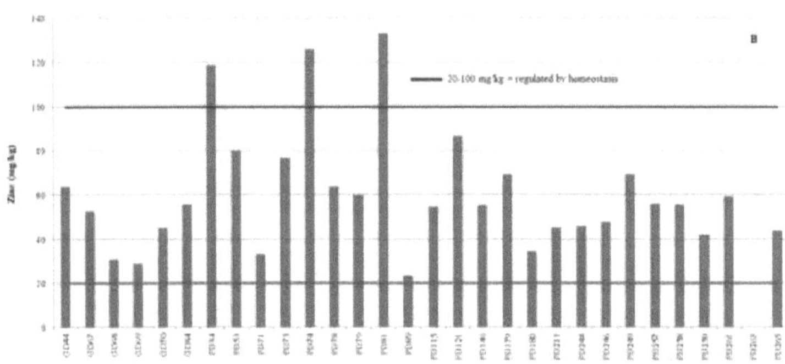

Figure 30 displays the levels of zinc (Zn) found in the liver of individual bottlenose dolphins

An investigation into the impact of biological and environmental factors on trace element concentrations through regression analysis yielded significant findings. This paper established that the year, which the dolphins had stranded, had a great influence on the amount of copper (Cu) and zinc (Zn) in their body tissues.

In addition, the geographical area of the strandings also affected the traces levels of these elements. Particularly, dolphins found in the south showed significantly fewer levels of Cu in muscle tissue than dolphins found in the north ($p = 0.049$, $b = 0.803$).

The Distribution of Copper Levels in Various Tissues

An example of this is seen in bottlenose dolphins of the Ligurian Sea, which had a concentration of copper of between 5.45 to 23.78mg/kg and a mean concentration of 14.61mg/kg.

On the same note, dolphins in Israel had concentrations ranging between 1 to 30mg/kg with an average of 11.4-11.8mg/kg.

Another species that showed high concentrations of copper in the liver was the striped dolphin with a level of 11.8 mg/kg which was similar to what is being recorded off-shore Israel and thus surpasses the normal levels of copper (<10 mg/kg) observed in the area.

The differences in these interspecies can be explained by the variability that exists in the diet, physiology, and ecology [418- 430].

Regarding kidney copper levels, it has been shown that there are considerable inter-species diversities ($p < 0.05$). Bottlenose dolphins had the highest renal levels of 6.26 0 -1 kg -1, followed by striped dolphins with 5.43 0 -1 kg -1 and Risso dolphins with 3.52 0 -1 kg -1.

Males exhibit a little greater concentration (6.05mg kg -1) than females (4.56mg kg -1). Renal copper levels in bottlenose dolphins were similar to those in Ligurian Sea but lower than those of Texas (12 0mg/kg -1) and southern Australia (7.35 0mg/kg -1). Markedly, copper levels of keyneys in striped dolphins were continually higher than those in the earlier Mediterranean studies that might be indicative of regional variations in exposure/retention [436, 441].

The pulmonary copper concentrations of bottlenose dolphins depended on age and sex with the highest level among a young male. Adult males, juveniles, and adult females had similar concentrations as compared to striped and Risso dolphins, which had significantly lower concentrations. In bottlenose dolphins the concentrations were generally high (similar to the reported concentrations in Corsica) but higher than those found in most of the other Mediterranean areas.

Limited data is available for spleen, skin, and adipose tissue copper concentrations in the Mediterranean. In this study, spleen copper concentrations were higher across all species compared to previous records. For skin copper levels, bottlenose dolphins had higher values compared to Corsica, Israel, and were comparable to Portugal, but lower compared to the peak average reported in Israel.

Striped dolphin skin copper levels aligned with Atlantic data from Portugal and exceeded most Mediterranean values. In adipose tissue, bottlenose dolphins had higher copper concentrations compared to Israel, while striped dolphins had lower levels compared to other Mediterranean studies. [**434**].

Age-Related Patterns

The research showed a clear-cut relationship between age and hepatic copper concentration. In the research, a juvenile bottlenose dolphin found in Apulia, Italy, had a very high concentration of hepatic copper of 80.65 mg/kg, though a juvenile with 19.34 mg/kg and an adult female with 8.29mg/kg were found in the same area. The decreasing copper level in the dolphin body with age is the same trend of striped dolphins in the French coastline, consequently indicating that there is a similarity in the trends of the various species and also in the geographical locations.

These elevated concentrations of hepatic copper in newborn dolphins have been well-known and they are attributed to the placental transfer of this mineral and their low ability to excrete copper in the early life. This buildup can be contributed to by the excessive synthesis of fetal metallothionein that helps in the storage of copper during pregnancy.

Since the mammalian milk has very little copper, the prenatal accumulation is necessary to sustain the growth after birth. It is also worth pointing out that copper regulation in cetaceans is generally highly regulated with the majority of alterations being experienced in the initial stages of the development. [**442- 452**].

Dietary Impact on Bioaccumulation

The accumulation of copper in organisms is greatly dependent on diet. The level of copper in the liver of dolphins at Risso, off the coast of Israel, was significantly high, but this can be attributed to the rich level of copper in their main food which is the cuttlefish (Sepia officinalis) that reaches 1450mg/kg.

Determination of the reference values is necessary to determine the possible toxicity of copper. Law et al. proposed a physiologically regulated range of hepatic copper 330 -1 wet weight. Any concentrations that are higher than this range signify that the homeostatic control is lost. It was discovered that a number of people, especially the juveniles, were above the top limit as shown in Figure 32, which necessitates more care of the vulnerable age groups and polluted surroundings. [**420- 424, 430**].

Factors Affecting Zinc Concentrations

The major deposition of zinc (Zn) in the integument of the marine mammals coincides with its known physiological functions in wound healing and protection against ultraviolet radiations. Empirical evidence has proved that Zn levels are significantly high in the superficial adipose layer than in deep strata, which has highlighted its significance in epidermal defense mechanisms.

When examining Zn levels in the skin of different dolphin species, those found in the Israeli coast had much higher levels as compared to those found in other Mediterranean areas. The skin tissue samples taken of dolphins in the current study showed Zn levels similar to the ones of dolphins in other areas and specifically high levels in bottle nose dolphins and striped dolphins along the Portuguese Atlantic coast. However, the amount of Zn in the skin of bottlenose dolphins in the Portuguese location measured in the period of another time frame was significantly less. The same patterns of fluctuation were witnessed in adipose tissue samples and different levels of Zn had been recorded in bottlenose dolphins at different times. [**434,**435].

The relationship between the concentration of zinc and the health condition of cetaceans is a scientific issue. Research has shown that increased concentrations of zinc in the liver result in a variety of diseases in these sea mammals. As an example, the harbor porpoises living in the coastal regions showed significantly elevated levels of zinc in liver tissue when they died of infectious diseases and not due to physical injuries [432].

A possible reason that could cause this effect is dietary factors; too much zinc or iron can inhibit the absorption of copper into the intestine by competitively inhibiting the absorption of copper at mucosal level which eventually results in the depletion of copper in the liver. [**457- 459**].

The results on French Mediterranean coast show that the amount of copper (Cu) and zinc (Zn) in the tissues of striped dolphins were within the same ranges of 2002 -2009. Equally, within the Eastern Mediterranean area, specifically the Levantine Basin, there were no significant variations in the concentration of copper, manganese (Mn), or zinc in bottlenose dolphins between 2004 to 2006, and in striped dolphins in Israel between 2001 and 2011.

However, there was a significant rise in the hepatic manganese levels between 2006 and 2011 as compared to 2001. These results are the implication that trace elements in the Mediterranean region are either stagnant or decreased over the last ten years. Wafo et al. [427], however, assert that, although there is a reduction in environmental contamination, there is no immediate or immediate effect on the reduction of the levels in marine organisms because of the cumulative nature of trace elements and its effects persistence. A detailed reading of about 20 years as was conducted in this paper gives a more accurate picture in terms of declining levels.

Comparison of copper levels in the livers of striped dolphins in the western Mediterranean and the Atlantic Ocean has shown no considerable difference. Stavros and others noticed a difference in the level of cobalt in the skin tissues of Florida and South Carolina bottlenose dolphins, highlighting the difference between regions.

Even though the lower concentrations of the trace elements caused by human activity are found in the Southern Hemisphere, marine fauna in the Southern

Hemisphere (Southern Ocean and the South Pole) show higher levels. The implication of these findings is that the trace elements in tissues might not be an effective measure of the extent of environmental pollution because bioavailability and diet have a higher impact on the trace element content in the tissues of marine mammals. [**462- 466**].

In the current research, there were no gender-specific variations in the trace element level, i.e. the level of copper and zinc, in any of the tissues. But as in the case of earlier studies, women were found to have much lower levels of manganese in the kidney as compared to their male counterparts ($p = 0.008$, $b = 0.850$) a fact also echoed by Monteiro et al. to the effect that gender differences do not have a significant influence on the levels of trace elements.

Copper in the lungs had a clear correlation with age ($p = 0.034$, $b = 0.968$) which showed a negative correlation with age. It is worth noting that the levels of copper and zinc were found to be high in younger people (fetuses and neonates) than adults. The findings are in agreement with previous research and support the idea that the fundamental trace elements accrue at stages of high tissue growth and cellular differentiation. The higher levels of copper and zinc in younger groups can be explained by the higher physiological needs and lower excretion especially in the fetal tissues.

Correlation between body length and mass and trace element levels in different tissues were evident though the levels differed among the elements. Copper in the kidney and adipose tissue, manganese in the kidney, liver, and adipose tissue, and zinc in the kidney in particular, decreased with the increase in body weight. On the other hand, the level of copper in the kidney and fatty tissues increased with the increase in body length. The implication of these findings is that metabolic control and element transport systems have a major effect on distribution of trace elements on tissues, overriding age or environmental exposure effects. [**454**].

Correlations among Levels of Trace Elements

Copper (Cu) and zinc (Zn) are crucial trace elements, which are a decisive part of the structure and enzymatic activity of numerous metalloenzymes. The levels of these components are controlled by metallothioneins an aggregate of small proteins, composed of cysteine, with high affinity to divalent metal ions.

Despite the previous research that proposed an interaction between Cu and Zn to be contradictory since they share the same regulation pathway, the current research combined with the one conducted by Lemos et al. has revealed that the correlation between the Cu and Zn levels is statistically significant, and positive. [470-472]

Concentration of protein in serum and the fractions of protein in serum

Serum protein electrophoresis (SPE) is used extensively and considered to be the valid method of investigating and measuring serum proteins. The approach is useful in clinical assessment as it can be used in conjunction with hematological and biochemical profiles to obtain valuable clinical data. The kinetics of total protein concentration, the dynamics of albumin and globulin fractions are more actively investigated in domestic and wild animals because of their characteristic patterns that can point to the immune, neoplastic, or inflammatory state.

Using the serum protein electrophoresis it is possible to identify the proteins in the serum by distinguishing between groups of proteins according to their migration velocities which depend on their size and electric charge. This separation is done in an electric field upon immobilizing the proteins on several surfaces, including agarose gel. As a result in the majority of domestic mammalian species, six distinct protein fractions have been differentiated based on their migration speeds and include albumin, 1, 2, 3, and 4 globulins. [473].

Unusual technologies are typically utilized to examine serum proteins in animals, and they include cellulose acetate electrophoresis (CAE) and agarose gel electrophoresis (AGE). Capillary zone electrophoresis (CZE) has also been popular in veterinary laboratories in recent years, because it has improved resolution of the peak of the electrophoresis, and it will process much faster and automatically. With these benefits, the high-cost nature of CZE is a constraint in the use of CZE in animals. The high-resolution electrophoresis technique, which is a means of isolating particular serum proteins, has been confirmed in dogs among the veterinary community and is scarcely accessible.

Serum total protein is commonly used as a diagnostic procedure that is critical to identifying and monitoring inflammatory conditions in several cetacean species including killer whales, minke whales, pantropical spotted dolphins, belugas and other marine mammals, including harbor seals and walruses. [**474- 482**].

A large number of research studies have shown the significance of evaluating the serum total protein as a salient and generally accepted indicator of inflammation. However, in the interpretation of clinical data, it is always necessary to pay special attention to specific analyzing techniques and reference ranges that are species-specific. When choosing a suitable reference group, various biological factors should also be considered and these include age, sex, and physiological factors including pregnancy.

In addition, in marine mammals, the environmental factors, natural or introduced by humans, are to be taken into account, specifically with individuals in the care of humans and which live in a restricted environment with limited exposure to pathogens [483-490].

The research used thirty-six samples, including eighteen cases of females and eighteen cases of males; nevertheless, two samples, one male and one female, were not included in the study since they had severe hemolysis conditions, and the electropherogram interpretation was not possible. Four major protein fractions (albumin, 0 -globulins, 0 -globulins, and 0 -globulins) were observed in each subject in the resultant cohort and a normal pattern was observed in all serum specimens without signs of a particular disease state.

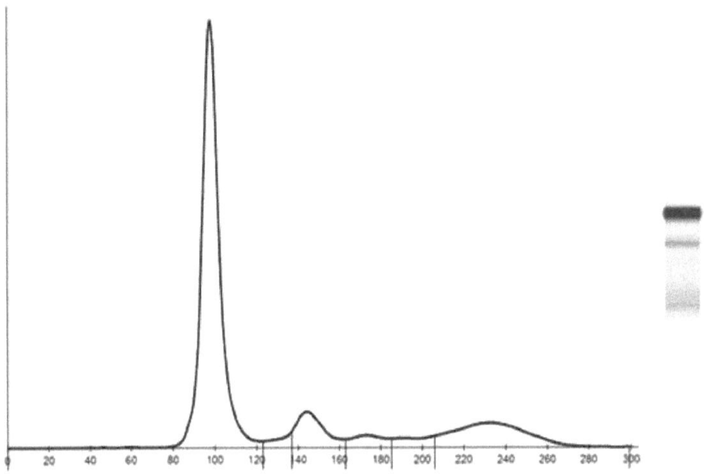

In Figure 31, the illustration of a serum protein electropherogram was on an agarose gel with special attention to bottlenose dolphins.

The intra-assay precision was found to be between 1.2 and 3.8 per cent. with regard to albumin and 2.5 to 5.7 per cent. with regard to α-globulins respectively.

After carrying out the Tukey test on the data, the percentage of γ -globulins had a single outlier value, which was then deleted. On the other hand, nine values, which are potential outliers were included in the dataset.

There were no statistically significant differences in the results of male and female dolphins related to total protein, all subfractions of serum protein (in percentages and concentration), and the ratio albumin/globulin with p -values of 0.32 to 0.98. Age distribution of the animals was categorised as follows: 10 animals were in the group of 1-11, 9 in the group of 12-17, 10 in the group of 18-23 and 9 in the group of 29-51.

No significant differences were discovered between the measured parameters with a level of significance ranging between P = -0.068 albumin g L -1 to P = -0.81 alpha -globulin g L -1. Box plots and histograms to indicate the distribution of the data are presented in Figure 35 and Figure 36.

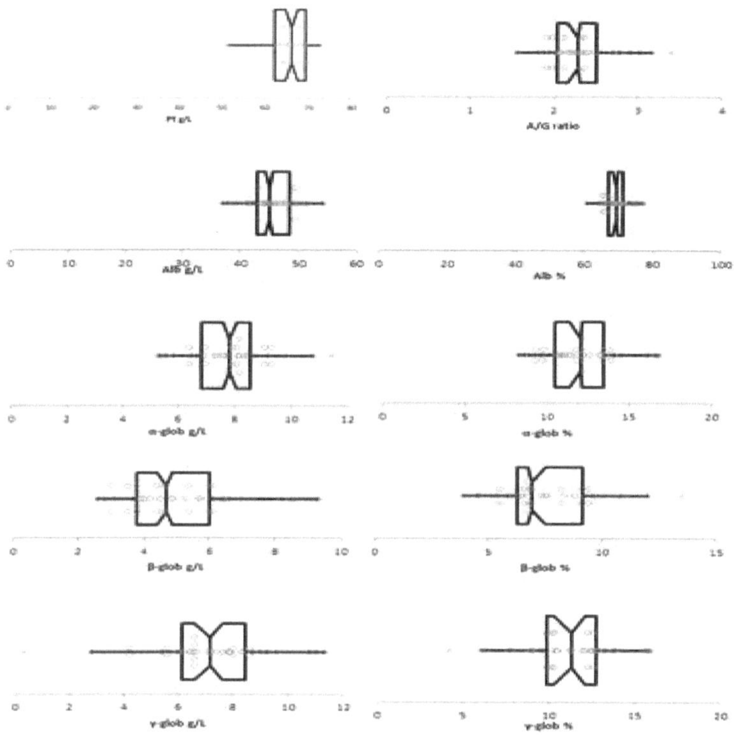

Figure 32 shows a boxplot of the information regarding different parameters of the protein, including total protein, the albumin to globulin ratio, and the albumin concentration in gram per liter and percentage.

In veterinary medicine, serum protein electrophoresis is regularly used to measure the concentrations of albumin and globulins, as this allows detection of changes in concentration that could be an indicator of inflammatory or infectious disease.

A study of total protein, albumin and globulin kinetics is increasingly becoming a focus of marine mammal research, due to the similarity of the pathology patterns that are experienced in terrestrial mammals and inflammatory states.

In mammals, 1/2 -globulins consist of 1/2-acid glycoprotein and haptoglobin; 2/3 -globulins consist of transferrin and serum amyloid-A; and 4-globulins consist of IgG and C-reactive protein.[490492].

Serum protein electrophoresis (SPE) is an excellent analytical method, which, though does not quantify individual proteins with an exception of albumin, can be used to quantify groups of proteins that have similar electrophoretic mobilities. The technique is very admired both in regular medical examinations and in clinical setting.

SPE is a relatively inexpensive method of assessing the progression of a disease quickly. Specifically, it helps to evaluate the health conditions, observe how the therapeutic exercise benefits healthy animals, and keep track of their recovery before being released into the environment.

The increasing endangered the marine mammals due to the pathogens like the Morbillivirus, Brucella ceti and Toxoplasma gondii which is why to understand the interactions between the host-specific pathogens and the marine mammals, analysis of the serum proteins fractions and identification of specific patterns is necessary.

Though acute-phase proteins (APPs) are sensitive indicators of inflammation, their cross-reactivity has been found to be limited to all proteins that can be found in marine mammals. In addition, there are usually species-specific reagents that are unavailable. This resource shortage further highlights the need to employ the serum protein electrophoresis (SPE) to gain a better insight into the health and well-being of marine mammals. [**495**].

Recent developments in procedures including high-resolution electrophoresis have improved the identification and separation of single proteins; the procedures have worked in dogs, but have yet to be utilized in marine mammals. Modern day capillary zone electrophoresis (CZE) has outperformed the age old agarose gel electrophoresis (AGE) techniques due to its high resolution.

The resolution that CZE offers in human and veterinary medicine is high enough to enable the minimization of the variation in analysis as well as increasing sensitivity in terms of identifying protein subfractions. Accordingly, these capacities enhance the likelihood of detecting atypical appearance of non-domesticated species or detecting abnormalities [496-498].

Setting the right reference limits in the interpretation of clinical and pathological data is necessary not only with regard to the species and methods used to measure the data but also taking into account the living conditions of the animals. Although CZE has benefits, its relatively high price has limited its implementation into the veterinary laboratory system and its application in non-domestic animals [499].

Moreover, the article by Schwacke and others on the free-ranging bottlenose dolphins did not filter possible unhealthy animals, which can have accounted to the given reference intervals. In comparison, we used dolphin serum samples in our study that had no reported clinical histories and complete physical examination.

Not only that, but a plethora of variables has been reported to affect clinical-pathological information, among them the environmental factors, gender, age, seasonal changes, etc., especially in non-domestic animals, as to reptiles and birds [501-503]. The current research has a small sample size that has restrained the further classification of the reference intervals in terms of age. The need to use 120 reference individuals complicates the assessment of non-domestic animals since 120 individuals are believed to be the best numbers that can be used to determine reference intervals. However, we used 38 reference individuals and it was enough to establish reference intervals.

Such periods, together with already published data, could be used as a basis of the interpretation of hematological and biochemical values in this particular species. Another solution, which is potentially successful in the context of restricted reference animals, is the creation of individualized reference intervals (iRIs). [504]

CONCLUSIONS

The use of animal models is essential in the explanation of the processes behind human diseases and the effectiveness of treatment measures. This implies that animal models need to be characterized accurately and validated as alternatives to human disease phenotypes as important to translational research. Out of the many animal models, the murine models are of specific significance in the study of human pathologies whereby pathology forms a critical endpoint in assessing and supporting these models.

The common sense in translational research is to be careful in all the stages of the model development and review since there are many crucial aspects to be considered when pathological analysis is conducted.

The developments in the field are vital in the diagnosis and treatment of the diseases affecting domestic and wild animals, and it is central to the health of people particularly concerning zoonotic diseases. Integration of new technologies and multidisciplinary and teamwork approaches will make the development of veterinary pathology decisive. Faced with such issues like new diseases and ethical concerns, a creative and active approach is needed.

Veterinary pathology is a vigilant and essential discipline, in constant flux and flux, and with a unique resolve to lifelong learning and change so that it may meet emerging illnesses and technology to benefit the animals and their health of the world.

The existing veterinary textbooks have an unclear definition of health and disease. Five categories can be separated in the definitions of health but they cannot be strictly related to some medical paradigms, including conventional or alternative veterinary medicine. An extended theoretical discussion of health and disease in veterinary medicine would go a long way in enhancing the field.

The seasonality and composition of feed are environmental conditions that cause a strong impact on the hematological indices, blood parameters, and mass of Creole goats, which demonstrate complex interactions. Diets should be adapted to meet current environmental conditions to effectively relieve the climatic stress on the tropical livestock system; protein-balanced diet improves metabolic and immunologic responses and leads to efficiency and sustainability.

In vitro organoid models of the ileal crypts of East Friesian sheep have been established successfully with a faithfully reproduced gastrointestinal structure and dynamics of the ovine species.

Sepsis is a serious complication and a health risk to both human and equine patients, which requires serious care and results in high expenses. Although the attention to new therapeutic interventions continues, supportive therapy is the most common one. The problems of sepsis management include disparities in personal immune system responses, selection of eligible targets to receive targeted therapies, and the ability to convert preclinical outcomes to clinical therapy. A universal definition of sepsis in the equine community can simplify the process of clinical trials by overcoming the issue associated with the complications of the inclusion criteria and facilitating the determination of the at-risk group. Monoclonal antibody therapy of equine sepsis is prohibitive in cost because of volumetric considerations and, therefore, hemoperfusion is potentially cost-effective. More studies are needed to optimize the cytokine modulation approaches in different groups of patients.

It is not defined which is the optimal level of cytokine elimination in sepsis patients that will be sufficient in balancing the defence against pathogen and safety of organs. Further research is required to gain an in-depth insight into the mechanisms of dysregulation of cytokines during sepsis as well as the optimization of cytokines modulation models. The alterations to transcutaneous auricular vagus nerve stimulation (tAVNS) parameters might be necessary to enhance the tolerability of horses and support the effectiveness of this technique to gastrointestinal disorders.

Composition of the expansion media influences the phenotype of the porcine myoblasts with the use of a mixture of fetal bovine serum (FBS) and basic fibroblast growth factor (bFGF) being favorable over horse serum. Isolation methods have little effects, and expansion procedures have significant effects on myoblast phenotype. To this end, it is suggested that when making samples of the skeletal muscle, porcine myoblasts should be obtained using young donors, grown under specific expansion conditions, and then cloned into CD56-expressing cells.

Differences in the levels of trace elements with age, sex, geographical origin make it hard to define the baseline of copper and zinc in dolphins, hence the need to include demographic and environmental factors in subsequent studies. The current investigation provides essential information on the metal levels of Adriatic dolphins, which helped to explain spatial, temporal and biological factors of metal concentration on these marine predators, and have implications to environmental surveillance and management practices. A larger sample size in future studies will enable establishment of reference ranges of captive bottlenose dolphins which are stratified by age and sex.

References

1. Jajosky RP, Brown M. The medical student's guide to pathology residency, fellowships, and careers. Ann Diagn Pathol. 2021;54:151805.
2. Soriano E, Pujadas L. Reelin reverts biochemical, physiological and cognitive alterations in mouse models of Tauopathy. Prog Neurobiol.2020;186:101743
3. Handy RD, Smith CJ. Toxicity of single walled carbon nanotubes to rainbow trout, (Oncorhynchus mykiss): Respiratory toxicity, organ pathologies, and other physiological effects. Aquat Toxicol. 2007;82:94-109.
4. Nicholls D, Perry G. The complexities of the pathology–pathogenesis relationship in Alzheimer disease. Biochem Pharmacol. 2014;88:671-676.
5. Valli T, Barthold SW, Ward JE, et al. Over 60% of NIH extramural funding involves animal-related research. Vet Pathol. 2007;44:962–963.
6. DeVoss J, Diehl L. Murine models of inflammatory bowel disease (IBD): Challenges of modeling human disease. Toxicol Pathol. 2014;42:99–110.
7. Ward JM, Schofield PN, Sundberg JP. Reproducibility of histopathological findings in experimental pathology of the mouse: A sorry tail. Lab Anim. 2017;46:146–151.
8. Cardiff RD, Rosner A, Hogarth MA, Galvez JJ, Borowsky AD, Gregg JP. Validation: The new challenge for pathology. Toxicol Pathol. 2004;32(Suppl. 1):31–39.
9. Cardiff RD, Ward JM, Barthold SW. _One medicine—one pathology': Are veterinary and human pathology prepared? Lab Invest. 2008;88:18–26.
10. Elmore SA, Peddada SD. Points to consider on the statistical analysis of rodent cancer bioassay data when incorporating historical control data. Toxicol Pathol. 2009;37:672–676.

11. Workman P, Aboagye EO, Balkwill F, et al. Guidelines for the welfare and use of animals in cancer research. Br J Cancer. 2010;102:1555–1577.
12. Kilkenny C, Browne WJ, Cuthill IC, Emerson M, Altman DG. Improving bioscience research reporting: The ARRIVE guidelines for reporting animal research. PLoS Biol. 2010;8:e1000412.
13. Falls T, Roy DG, Bell JC, Bourgeois-Daigneault MC. Murine tumor models for oncolytic rhabdovirotherapy. ILAR J. 2016;57:73–85.
14. Scudamore CL, Soilleux EJ, Karp NA, et al. Recommendations for minimum information for publication of experimental pathology data: MINPEPA guidelines. J Pathol. 2016;238:359–367.
15. National Research Council (US) Institute for Laboratory Animal Research Guidance for the Description of Animal Research in Scientific Publications. Washington, DC: National Academies Press (US); 2011.
16. Zeiss CJ, Ward JM, Allore HG. Designing phenotyping studies for genetically engineered mice. Vet Pathol. 2012;49:24–31.
17. Justice MJ, Siracusa LD, Stewart F. Technical approaches for mouse models of human disease. Dis Model Mech. 2011;4:305–310.
18. Sellers RS. The gene or not the gene—That is the question: Understanding the genetically engineered mouse phenotype. Vet Pathol. 2011;49:5–15.
19. Higashi AY, Ikawa T, Muramatsu M, et al. Direct hematological toxicity and illegitimate chromosomal recombination caused by the systemic activation of CreER^{T2}. J Immunol. 2009;182:5633–5640.
20. Sellers RS, Clifford CB, Treuting PM, Brayton C. Immunological variation between inbred laboratory mouse strains: Points to consider in phenotyping genetically immunomodified mice. Vet Pathol. 2012;49:32–43.

21. Brayton CF, Treuting PM, Ward JM. Pathobiology of aging mice and GEM: Background strains and experimental design. Vet Pathol. 2012;49:85–105.
22. Haines DC, Chattopadhyay S, Ward JM. Pathology of aging B6; 129 mice. Toxicol Pathol. 2001;29:653–661.
23. Sellers RS. Translating mouse models: Immune variation and efficacy testing. Toxicol Pathol. 2017;45:134–145.
24. Szymanska H, Lechowska-Piskorowska J, Krysiak E, et al. Neoplastic and nonneoplastic lesions in aging mice of unique and common inbred strains contribution to modeling of human neoplastic diseases. Vet Pathol. 2014;51:663–679.
25. Bult CJ, Krupke DM, Eppig JT. Electronic access to mouse tumor data: The Mouse Tumor Biology Database (MTB) project. Nucleic Acids Res. 1999;27:99–105.
26. Brayton C, Justice M, Montgomery CA. Evaluating mutant mice: Anatomic pathology. Vet Pathol. 2001;38:1–19.
27. Barthold SW. Genetically altered mice: Phenotypes, no phenotypes, and faux phenotypes. Genetica. 2004;122:75–88.
28. Justice MJ, Dhillon P. Using the mouse to model human disease: Increasing validity and reproducibility. Dis Model Mech. 2016;9:101–103.
29. Barthold SW. ―Muromics": Genomics from the perspective of the laboratory mouse. Comp Med. 2002;52:206–223.
30. Linder CC. Mouse nomenclature and maintenance of genetically engineered mice. Comp Med. 2003;53:119–125.
31. Sundberg JP, Schofield PN. Commentary: Mouse genetic nomenclature. Standardization of strain, gene, and protein symbols. Vet Pathol. 2010;47:1100–1104.

32. Wotjak CT. C57BLack/BOX? The importance of exact mouse strain nomenclature. Trends Genet. 2003;19:183–184.
33. Lai Y, Wei X, Lin S, Qin L, Cheng L, Li P. Current status and perspectives of patient-derived xenograft models in cancer research. J Hematol Oncol. 2017;10:106.
34. Nakai N, Kawaguchi C, Nawa K, et al. Detection and elimination of contaminating microorganisms in transplantable tumors and cell lines. Exp Anim. 2000;49:309–313.
35. Manuel CA, Bagby SM, Reisinger JA, et al. A horizontal transfer technique of PDX tumors to eliminate Corynebacterium bovis. J Am Assoc Lab Anim Sci. 2017;56:166–172.
36. Treuting PM, Snyder JM, Ikeno Y, Schofield PN, Ward JM, Sundberg JP. The vital role of pathology in improving reproducibility and translational relevance of aging studies in rodents. Vet Pathol. 2016;53:244–249.
37. Bolon B, Barthold SW, Boyd KL, et al. Gender agenda: Sex bias can be justified in animal research. Nature. 2010;466:28.]
38. Treuting PM, Clifford CB, Sellers RS, Brayton CF. Of mice and microflora: Considerations for genetically engineered mice. Vet Pathol. 2012;49:44–63.
39. Burkholder T, Foltz C, Karlsson E, Linton CG, Smith JM. Health evaluation of experimental laboratory mice. Curr Protoc Mouse Biol. 2012;2:145–165.
40. 36. Traslavina RP, King EJ, Loar AS, et al. Euthanasia by CO2 inhalation effects potassium levels in mice. J Am Assoc Lab Anim Sci. 2010;49:316–322.
41. Schnell MA, Hardy C, Hawley M, Propert KJ, Wilson JM. Effect of blood collection technique in mice on clinical pathology parameters. Hum Gene Ther. 2002;13:155–162.

42. O‘Connell KE, Mikkola AM, Stepanek AM, et al. Practical murine hematopathology: A comparative review and implications for research. Comp Med. 2015;65:96–113.
43. McGarry MP, Protheroe CA, Lee JJ. Mouse Hematology: A Laboratory Manual. Cold Spring Harbor, NY: Cold Spring Harbor Laboratory Press; 2010.
44. Reagan WJ, Irizarry-Rovira A, Poitout-Belissent F, et al. Best practices for evaluation of bone marrow in nonclinical toxicity studies. Vet Clin Pathol. 2011;40:119–134.
45. Ward JM, Rehg JE. Rodent immunohistochemistry: Pitfalls and troubleshooting. Vet Pathol. 2014;51:8–101.
46. Goodwin PC, Johnson B, Frevert CW. Microscopy, immunohistochemistry, digital imaging, and quantitative microscopy In: Treuting PM, Dintzis SM, eds. Comparative Anatomy and Histology: A Mouse, Rat, and Human Atlas. 2nd ed London: Academic Press; 2018:53–66.
47. Knoblaugh SE, Randolph-Habecker J. Necropsy and histology In: Treuting PM, Dintzis SM, eds. Comparative Anatomy and Histology: A Mouse, Rat, and Human Atlas. 2nd ed London: Academic Press; 2018:23–51.
48. Treuting PM, Snyder JM. Mouse necropsy. Curr Protoc Mouse Biol. 2015;5:223–233.
49. Parkinson CM, O‘Brien A, Albers TM, Simon MA, Clifford CB, Pritchett-Corning KR. Diagnostic necropsy and selected tissue and sample collection in rats and mice. J Vis Exp. 2011;54:2966.
50. Ward JM, Treuting PM. Rodent intestinal epithelial carcinogenesis: Pathology and preclinical models. Toxicol Pathol. 2014;42:148–161

51. Shappell SB, Thomas GV, Roberts RL, et al. Prostate pathology of genetically engineered mice: Definitions and classification. The consensus report from the Bar Harbor meeting of the Mouse Models of Human Cancer Consortium Prostate Pathology Committee. Cancer Res. 2004;64:2270–2305.
52. Ittmann M, Huang J, Radaelli E, et al. Animal models of human prostate cancer: The consensus report of the New York meeting of the Mouse Models of Human Cancers Consortium Prostate Pathology Committee. Cancer Res. 2013;73:2718–2736.
53. 49. Suwa T, Nyska A, Haseman JK, Mahler JF, Maronpot RR. Spontaneous lesions in control B6C3F1 mice and recommended sectioning of male accessory sex organs. Toxicol Pathol. 2002;30:228–234.
54. Cardiff RD, Anver MR, Gusterson BA, et al. The mammary pathology of genetically engineered mice: The consensus report and recommendations from the Annapolis meeting. Oncogene. 2000;19:968–988.
55. Ruehl-Fehlert C, Kittel B, Morawietz G, et al. Revised guides for organ sampling and trimming in rats and mice—Part 1. Exp Pathol. 2003;55:91–106.
56. Kittel B, Ruehl-Fehlert C, Morawietz G, et al. Revised guides for organ sampling and trimming in rats and mice—Part 2. Exp Toxicol Pathol. 2004;55:413–431.
57. Morawietz G, Ruehl-Fehlert C, Kittel B, et al. Revised guides for organ sampling and trimming in rats and mice—Part 3. Exp Toxicol Pathol. 2004;55:433–449.
58. Latendresse JR, Warbrittion AR, Jonassen H, Creasy DM. Fixation of testes and eyes using a modified Davidson‘s fluid: Comparison with Bouin‘s fluid and conventional Davidson‘s fluid. Toxicol Pathol. 2002;30:524–533.

59. Brayton CF, Treuting PM. Phenotyping In: Treuting PM, Dintzis SM, eds. Comparative Anatomy and Histology: A Mouse, Rat, and Human Atlas. 2nd ed London: Academic Press; 2018:9–21.
60. Bolon B, La Perle KMD. Principles of experimental design for mouse developmental pathology studies In: Bolon B. (Ed.). Pathology of the Developing Mouse: A Systematic Approach. Boca Raton, FL: CRC Press (Taylor & Francis); 2015:117–132.
61. Bolon B, Newbigging S, Boyd KL. Pathology evaluation of developmental phenotypes in neonatal and juvenile mice. Curr Protoc Mouse Biol. 2017;7:191–219.
62. Rao DB, Little PB, Malarkey DE, Sills RC. Histopathological evaluation of the nervous system in National Toxicology Program rodent studies: A modified approach. Toxicol Pathol. 2011;39:463–470.
63. Meyerholz DK, Sieren JC, Beck AP, Flaherty HA. Approaches to evaluate lung inflammation in translational research. Vet Pathol. 2018;55:42–52.
64. Keenan CM, Baker J, Bradley A, et al. International Harmonization of Nomenclature and Diagnostic Criteria (INHAND): Progress to date and future plans. Toxicol Pathol. 2015;28:51–53.
65. Cardiff RD, Anver MR, Boivin GP, et al. Precancer in mice: Animal models used to understand, prevent, and treat human precancers. Toxicol Pathol. 2006;34:699–707.
66. Ward J. Preneoplastic and precancerous lesions in rodents: Morphologic and molecular characteristics. J Toxicol Pathol. 2002;15:123–128.
67. Frese KK, Tuveson DA. Maximizing mouse cancer models. Nat Rev Cancer. 2007;7:645–658.

68. Boivin GP, Washington K, Yang K, et al. Pathology of mouse models of intestinal cancer: Consensus report and recommendations. Gastroenterology. 2003;124:762–777.
69. Nikitin AY, Alcaraz A, Anver MR, et al. Classification of proliferative pulmonary lesions of the mouse: Recommendations of the Mouse Models of Human Cancers Consortium. Cancer Res. 2004;64:2307–2316
70. 66. Hruban RH, Adsay NV, Albores-Saavedra J, et al. Pathology of genetically engineered mouse models of pancreatic exocrine cancer: Consensus report and recommendations. Cancer Res. 2006;66:95–106.
71. Washington MK, Powell AE, Sullivan R, et al. Pathology of rodent models of intestinal cancer: Progress report and recommendations. Gastroenterology. 2013;144:705–717.
72. McCormick F (2010) The molecular pathology of cancer. Nat Rev Clin Oncol 7:251–265
73. Pentimalli A, Giordano A. Cell biology and genetics. Life Sci. 2017. https://doi.org/10.1016/B978-0-12-809633-8.12390-8
74. Wagner HN (1995) Nuclear medicine: what it is and what it does. In: Wagner HN, Szabo Z, Buchanan JW (eds) Principles of nuclear medicine. Saunders, Philadelphia, pp 1–8
75. Virchow R (1958) Disease, life, and man. Stanford University Press, Stanford
76. McCance KL, Huether SE (2005) Pathophysiology. The biologic basis for disease in adults and children, 4th edn. Mosby, St. Louis
77. Cotran RS, Kumar V, Collins T (2010) Robbins pathologic basis of disease, 8th edn. Saunders, Philadelphia
78. Pollard TD, Earnshaw WC (2002) Cell biology. Saunders, Philadelphia

79. Wobeser GA. Essentials of disease in wild animals. John Wiley & Sons; 2013.
80. Simpson VR. Wild animals as reservoirs of infectious diseases in the UK. The Veterinary Journal. 2002;163(2):128-146.
81. Sharma AK, Nayakwadi S, Chandratre GA, Saini M, Das A, Raut SS, Somvanshi R. Prevalence of pathological conditions in zoo/wild animals in India: a retrospective study based on necropsy. Proceedings of the National Academy of Sciences, India Section B: Biological Sciences. 2014;84: 937-946.
82. Singh AK, Yadav N, Singh A, Singh A. Transcription factors that regulate gene expression under drought. In Acta Biology Forum. 2023;2:01-04.
83. Bercovier H, Vincent V. Mycobacterial infections in domestic and wild animals due toMycobacterium marinum. Rev. sci. tech. Off. int. Epiz. 2001;20(1):265-290.
84. Youssef SA, Capucchio MT, Rofina JE, Chambers JK, Uchida K, Nakayama H, Head E. Pathology of the aging and animal models of human neurodegenerative diseases. Veterinary Pathology 2016;53(2):327-348.
85. Maxie G. Jubb, Kennedy & Palmer's pathology of domestic animals. 2015;2(2). Elsevier health sciences.
86. Seyedmousavi S, Guillot J, Arné P, De Hoog GS, Mouton JW, Melchers WJ, Verweij PE. Aspergillus and aspergilloses in wild and domestic animals: a global health concern with parallels to human disease. Medical Mycology. 2015;53(8): 765-797.
87. Gavier-Widén D, Meredith A, Duff JP (Eds.). Infectious Diseases of wild Mammals and birds in Europe. John Wiley & Sons; 2012.

88. Coelho AC, de Lurdes Pinto M, Matos A, Matos M, dos Anjos Pires M. Mycobacterium avium complex in domestic and wild animals. In Insights from veterinary medicine. InTechOpen; 2013.
89. Mydeen AKM, Agnihotri N, Bahadur R, Lytand W, Kumar N, Hazarika S. Microbial Maestros: Unraveling the crucial role of microbes in shaping the Environment. In Acta Biology Forum. 2023;2:23-28.
90. Emikpe BO, Morenikeji OA, Jarikre TA. Zoo animals' disease pattern in a university zoological garden, Ibadan, Nigeria. Asian Pacific Journal of Tropical Disease. 2016;6(2):85-89.
91. Brioudes, Aurélie, Jeffrey Warner, Robert Hedlefs, and Bruce Gummow. A review of domestic animal diseases within the Pacific Islands region. Acta Tropica. 2014; 132:23-38.
92. Fowler ME, Miller ER. Zoo and Wild Animal Medicine Current Therapy-E-Book. Elsevier Health Sciences; 2007.
93. Singh CD. Advanced pathology and treatment of diseases of domestic animals. International Book Distributing Co., Lucknow. 2008;87-89.
94. Sikkander AM. Duct cancer evaluation in situ–review. In Acta Biology Forum. 2022; 01-04.
95. Feldman WH. Neoplasms of domesticated animals. Neoplasms of Domesticated Animals; 1932.
96. Siso S, Hanzlicek D, Fluehmann G, Kathmann I, Tomek A, Papa V, Vandevelde M. Neurodegenerative diseases in domestic animals: a comparative review. The Veterinary Journal. 2006;171(1):20-38.
97. Junginger, Johannes, Florian Hansmann, Vanessa Herder, Annika Lehmbecker, Martin Peters, Martin Beyerbach, Peter Wohlsein, and

Wolfgang Baumgärtner. "Pathology in captive wild felids at German zoological gardens. PLoS One. 201510(6): e0130573.

98. Woodford MH. Veterinary aspects of ecological monitoring: the natural history of emerging infectious diseases of humans, domestic animals and wildlife. Tropical animal health and production. 2009;41(7): 1023-1033.

99. van Asten AJ, Nikolaou GN, Gröne A. The occurrence of cpb2-toxigenic Clostridium perfringens and the possible role of the β2-toxin in enteric disease of domestic animals, wild animals and humans. The Veterinary Journal. 2010;183(2):135-140.

100. Lempp C, Jungwirth N, Grilo ML, Reckendorf A, Ulrich A, Van Neer A, Siebert U. Pathological findings in the red fox (*Vulpes vulpes*), stone marten (*Martes foina*) and raccoon dog *(Nyctereutes procyonoides*), with special emphasis on infectious and zoonotic agents in Northern Germany. PLoS One. 2017;12(4): e0175469.

101. Pope Jenny P, Debra L, Miller, Matthew C. Riley. Eman Anis, and Rebecca P. Wilkes. "Characterization of a novel canine distemper virus causing disease in wildlife. Journal of Veterinary Diagnostic Investigation. 2016;28(5):506-513.

102. Radostits OM, Gay C, Hinchcliff KW, Constable PD. (Eds.). Veterinary Medicine E-Book: A textbook of the diseases of cattle, horses, sheep, pigs and goats. Elsevier Health Sciences; 2006.

103. Stevenson DE, Wilson AA. Metabolic disorders of domestic animals. Metabolic disorders of Domestic Animals; 1963.

104. Shtrasburg S, Gal R, Gruys E, Perl S, Martin BM, Kaplan B, Livneh A. An ancillary tool for the diagnosis of amyloid A amyloidosis in a variety of domestic and wild animals. Veterinary Pathology. 2005; 42(2):132-139.

105. Hámori D. Constitutional disorders and hereditary diseases in domestic animals. Elsevier Scientific Publishing Company; 1983.

106. Ghosh D, Ekta Ghosh D. A Large-Scale Multi-Centre Research On Domain General-isation in Deep Learning-Based Mass Detection in Mammography: A Review. In Acta Biology Forum. 2022;05-09.

107. Ashokri HAA, Abuzririq MAK. The impact of environmental awareness on personal carbon footprint values of biology department students, Faculty of Science, El-Mergib University, Al-Khums, Libya. In Acta Biology Forum. 2023;18:22.

108. Francis J. Tuberculosis in animals and man. A study in comparative pathology. *Tuberculosis in animals and man.* A Study in Comparative Pathology; 1958.

109. Sikkander AM. Assess of hydrazine sulphate (N2H6SO4) in opposition for the majority of cancer cells. In Acta Biology Forum. 2022;10-13.

110. Berny PJ, Buronfosse T, Buronfosse F, Lamarque F, Lorgue G. Field evidence of secondary poisoning of foxes (*Vulpes vulpes*) and buzzards (*Buteo buteo*) by bromadiolone, a 4-year survey. Chemosphere. 1997;35(8):1817-1829.

111. Akhtar K, Ahmed I, Tipu MY, Yaqub T, Shahid M, ur Rehman A, Aslam A. Molecular identification and infection pathology of Mycobacterium spp. in captive wild animals in Pakistan. The Journal of Infection in Developing Countries. 2023;17(08):1107-1113.

112. Swabe J. Animals, disease and human society: human-animal relations and the rise of veterinary medicine. Routledge; 2002.

113. Ghosh D, Ekta Ghosh D. Intensive Training in Breast Imaging with Artificial Intel-ligence and Deep Learning-A Review Article. In Acta Biology Forum. 2022;18-26.
114. Martin SW, Meek AH, Willeberg P. Veterinary epidemiology: Principles and methods. Ames, Iowa, USA, Iowa State university press; 1987.
115. Broom DM. Animal Welfare Defined in Terms of Attempts to Cope with the Environment. Acta Agric Scand Sect A, Animal Sci Suppl. 1996;27:22–28.
116. Blood DC, Henderson JA. Veterinary medicine. 4. London, Baillière Tindall; 1974.
117. Blood DC, Henderson JA, Radostits OM. Veterinary medicine: A textbook of the diseases of cattle, sheep, pigs & horses. 5. London, Baillière Tindall; 1979.
118. Blood DC, Radostits OM. Veterinary medicine: A textbook of the diseases of cattle, sheep, pigs, goats & horses. 7. London, Baillière Tindall; 1989.
119. Radostits OM, Blood DC, Gay CC. Veterinary medicine: A textbook of the diseases of cattle, sheep, pigs, goats & horses. 8. London, Baillière Tindall; 1994.
120. Radostits OM, Gay CC, Blood DC, Hinchcliff KW. Veterinary medicine: A textbook of the diseases of cattle, sheep, pigs, goats & horses. 9. London, Baillière Tindall; 2000.
121. Geyer G, Grabner A. Die Tierarzthelferin; Leitfaden für den Fachkundeunterricht der Tierarzthelferin; Kurzgefasster Ratgeber für Tierarztfrauen und Helfer in der Praxis. 1. Schlütersche Verlagsanstalt und Druckerei; 1983.
122. Geyer G, Grabner A. Die Tierarzthelferin; Leitfaden für den Fachkundeunterricht der Tierarzthelferin; Kurzgefasster Ratgeber für

Tierarztfrauen und Helfer in der Praxis. 3. Schlütersche Verlagsanstalt und Druckerei; 1988.

123. Geyer G, Grabner A. Die Tierarzthelferin; Leitfaden für den Fachkundeunterricht der Tierarzthelferin; Kurzgefasster Ratgeber für Tierarztfrauen und Helfer in der Praxis. 4. Schlütersche Verlagsanstalt und Druckerei; 1991.
124. Brock K, Nielsen J. Veterinær homøopati – En indføring i homøopatisk diagnostik og terapi på dyr. København, DSR Forlag Landbohøjskolen; 1986.
125. Day C. The homeopathic treatment of beef & dairy cattle. Beaconsfield, Bucks, England, Beaconsfield publishers Ltd; 1995.
126. Thoresen AS. Veterinærmedisin alternative metoder – funksjonell veterinærmedisin med grunnlag i en helhetlig anskuelse. Oslo; 1997.
127. Blood DC, Studdert VP. Baillière's Comprehensive Veterinary Dictionary. 1. London, Baillière Tindall; 1988.
128. Blood DC, Studdert VP. Saunders comprehensive veterinary dictionary. 2. London, WB Saunders; 1999.
129. Thomson RG. Special veterinary pathology. Toronto, BC Decker Inc; 1988.
130. Ettinger SJ, Feldman EC. Textbook of veterinary internal medicine: diseases of the dog and cat. 5. 1&2. Philadelphia, WB Saunders company; 2000.
131. FAO. Manual for animal health auxiliary personnel. Rome, Food & Agriculture Organization of the United Nations; 1983.
132. Webster J. Understanding the dairy cow. Worcester, Great Britain, BSP Professional Books; 1987.
133. Wiesner E, Ribbeck R. Wörterbuch der Veterinärmedizin. 2. Stuttgart, Gustav Fischer Verlag; 1983.

134. Arnall L, Keymer IF. Bird disease; an introduction to the study of birds in health & disease. London, t.f.h; 1975.
135. Baker JK, Greer WJ. Animal health: A layman's guide to disease control. Danville, Illinois, IPP The Interstate Printers & Publishers Inc; 1980.
136. Hoopes KH, Thwaits RN. Principles of veterinary science. Baltimore, USA, Williams & Wilkins; 1997.
137. Slauson DO, Cooper BJ. Mechanisms of disease: A textbook of comparative general pathology. 2. Baltimore, USA, Williams & Wilkins; 1990.
138. Gillespie JH, Timoney JF. Hagan and Bruner's infectious diseases of domestic animals; with reference to etiology, pathogenicity, immunity, epidemiology, diagnosis, and biologic therapy. 7. Itaca, N.Y., USA, Cornell University Press; 1981.
139. Cheville NF. Introduction to veterinary pathology. Ames, Iowa, Iowa State University Press; 1988.
140. Lagerlöf N, Hallgren W, Ekesbo I. Husdjurens hälso-och sjukvårdslära. (Handbook of animal health and animal care) 3. Stockholm, Sweden, LTs förlag; 1968.
141. Ekesbo I. Kompendium i husdjurshygien (Compendium in Animal Hygiene) 8. Skara, Sweden, Department of Animal Environment and Health, Swedish University of Agricultural Sciences (SLU); 2002.
142. Duncan IJH. Animal welfare defined in terms of feelings. Acta Agric Scand Sect A, Animal Sci Suppl. 1996;27:29–35.
143. Fraser D, Weary DM, Pajor EA, Milligan BN. A scientific conception of animal welfare that reflects ethical concerns. Animal Welfare. 1997;6:187–205.
144. West GP. Black's veterinary dictionary. 18. London, A&C Black; 1995.

145. Aspinall KW. First step in veterinary science. London, Baillière Tindall; 1976.
146. Sainsbury D. Farm animal welfare; Cattle, pigs & poultry. London, Collins; 1986.
147. Zapata-Campos, C.C.; Mellado-Bosque, M.Á. The goat: Selection and consumption habits of native plants in arid rangelands. *Cienc. UAT* **2021**, *15*, 169–185.
148. Gonzales Aparicio, G.W.; Gutiérrez Reynoso, G.A.; Ponce de León, F.A.; Chauca Francia, D. Hematological study of Creole and Brown Swiss cattle raised in the Andes of Peru. *J. Vet. Res. Peru* **2020**, *31*, e19032.
149. Vicente-Pérez, A.; Avendaño-Reyes, L.; Barajas-Cruz, R.; Macías-Cruz, U.; Correa-Calderón, A.; Vicente-Pérez, R.; Corrales-Navarro, J.L.; Guerra-Liera, J.E. Biochemical and hematological parameters in hair sheep with and without shade under desert conditions. *Ecosyst. Agric. Resour.* **2018**, *5*, 259–269.
150. García-Sánchez, H.D.; Castellanos-Pérez, E.; Gallegos-Robles, M.Á.; García-Hernández, J.L. Blood parameters of grazing goats at three physiological stages throughout the year. *Ecosistemas Recur. Agropecu.* **2023**, *10*, e3506.
151. Guzmán Medina, L.E.; Callacná Custodio, M.Á. Hematological values of Creole goats in two physiological reproductive states. *Sci. Agropecu.* **2013**, *4*, 285–292. Available online: **https://www.researchgate.net/publication/277907063_Hematological_values_of_creole_goats_in_two_reproductive_physiological_states** (accessed on 3 March 2025).

152. Ojeda Fermoselle, P.M.; Manes, J.; Aller, J.F. Seasonal variations in reproductive parameters, semen quality, and testosterone levels in Highlander rams. *J. Vet. Res. Peru* **2021**, *32*, e19788.

153. Cedeño, H.; Ríos, K.; Pile, E.; Saavedra, R.; Sánchez-Galán, E.; Pimentel, T.; Remy, G.; Grajales-Cedeño, J. Effect of breed, season, month and time on the physiological and productive responses of dairy goats in a humid tropical environment. *Semilla Este* **2023**, *4*, 166–191.

154. Fernández del Palacio, M.J.; Montes, A.M.; Gutiérrez Panizo, C.; Bayón, A.; Bernal, L.J.; Sotillo, J. Blood biochemical parameters in male goats of the Murciano-Granadina breed. *Ann. Vet. Med. Murcia* **1991**, *6-7*, 3–7. Available online: **https://revistas.um.es/analesvet/article/view/20191** (accessed on 3 March 2025).

155. García, R.D. Instruments that revolutionized chemistry: The history of the spectrophotometer. *Adv. Chem.* **2018**, *13*, 79–82. Available online: **https://www.redalyc.org/journal/933/93368279004/html/** (accessed on 3 March 2025).

156. R Core Team. *R: A Language and Environment for Statistical Computing*; R Foundation for Statistical Computing: Vienna, Austria, 2023; Available online: **https://www.scirp.org/reference/referencespapers?referenceid=3582659** (accessed on 3 March 2025).

157. Rodríguez, L.A.; Mantecón, A.R.; Lavín, P.; Asensio, C.; Martín-Diana, A.B.; Olmedo, S.; Khedim, M.B.; Delgado, D.; Pérez, A.R.; Bartolomé, D. *Hematological and Blood Biochemical Parameters in Assaf Breed Sheep and Lambs*; SEOC 2011; Agrarian Technological Institute of Castilla y León: Valladolid, Spain, 2011; Available online: **https://digital.csic.es/bitstream/10261/41750/3/Reg.%207%20Rodr**

iguez%2C%20L.%20A.%20SEOC%202011.pdf (accessed on 18 March 2025).

158. Zaher, H.A.; Alawaash, S.A.; Tolba, A.M.; Swelum, A.A.; Abd El-Hack, M.E.; Taha, A.E.; Abdelnour, S.A. Impacts of Moringa oleifera foliage substituted with concentrate feed on growth, nutrient digestibility, hematological attributes and blood minerals of growing goats under Abu Dhabi conditions. *Sustainability* **2020**, *12*, 6096.
159. Chávez-García, D.; Acosta-Lozano, N.; Andrade-Yucailla, V. Determination of hematological values in native goats supplemented with Moringa oleifera Lam located in the lowland deciduous forest. *Amaz. J. Sci. Technol.* **2019**, *8*, 180–191. Available online: **https://dialnet.unirioja.es/descarga/articulo/7153087.pdf** (accessed on 18 March 2025).
160. Souza, B.B.; Assis, D.Y.C.; Silva Neto, F.L.; Roberto, R.; Marques, B.A.A. Effect of climate and diet on physiological and hematological parameters of Saanen goats kept in confinement in the Paraíba backlands. *Green J. Agroecol. Sustain. Dev.* **2011**, *6*, 77–82. Available online: **https://dialnet.unirioja.es/servlet/articulo?codigo=7429765** (access ed on 18 March 2025).
161. Washaya, A.; Mupangwa, J.; Muchenje, V.; Mpendulo, C.T. Biochemical indices and hematological parameters of goats fed Lablab purpureus and Vigna unguiculata as supplements to a basal Chloris gayana diet. *Vet. Anim. Sci.* **2019**, *8*, 100073.
162. Ribeiro, N.L.; Costa, R.G.; Pimenta Filho, E.C.; Ribeiro, M.N.; Crovetti, A.; Saraiva, E.P.; Bozzi, R. Adaptive profile of Garfagnina goat breed assessed

through physiological, haematological, biochemical and hormonal parameters. *Small Rumin. Res.* **2016**, *144*, 236–241.

163. Ghosh, S.; Singh, A.K.; Haldar, C. Adaptive and ecological significance of seasonal changes in hematological, biochemical, and hormonal parameters in the tropical goat *Capra hircus*. *J. Endocrinol. Reprod.* **2013**, *17*, 113–122. Available online: **https://informaticsjournals.co.in/index.php/jer/article/view/1919** (accessed on 18 March 2025).
164. Piccione, G.; Casella, S.; Lutri, L.; Vazzana, I.; Ferrantelli, V.; Caola, G. Reference values for some hematological, hematochemical and electrophoretic parameters in the Girgentana goat. *Turk. J. Vet. Anim. Sci.* **2010**, *34*, 197–204.
165. Daramola, J.O.; Adeloye, A.A.; Fatoba, T.A.; Soladoye, A.O. Hematological and biochemical parameters of West African dwarf goats. *Livest. Res. Rural Dev.* **2005**, *17*, 95. Available online: **http://www.lrrd.org/lrrd17/8/dara17095.htm** (accessed on 18 March 2025).
166. Njidda, A.A.; Hassan, I.T.; Olatunji, E.A. Haematological and biochemical parameters of goats of semi-arid environment fed on natural grazing rangeland of Northern Nigeria. *J. Agric. Vet. Sci.* **2013**, *3*, 1–8. Available online: **https://www.researchgate.net/publication/314540765_Haematological_and_Biochemical_Parameters_of_Goats_of_Semi_Arid_Environment_Fed_On_Natural_Grazing_Rangeland_of_Northern_Nigeria** (accessed on 21 March 2025).
167. Ahmed Mohammed, S.; Abdur Razzaque, M.; Omar, A.E.; Albert, S.; Al-Gallaf, W.M. Biochemical and hematological profile of different breeds of

goats maintained under intensive production system. *Afr. J. Biotechnol.* **2016**, *15*, 1253–1257. Available online: **https://www.ajol.info/index.php/ajb/article/view/140549** (accessed on 21 March 2025).

168. Olafadehan, O.A. Changes in hematological and biochemical diagnostic parameters of Red Sokoto goats fed tannin-rich *Pterocarpus erinaceus*. *Vet. Arch.* **2011**, *81*, 471–483.
169. Akkaya, F.; Senturk, S.; Mecitoğlu, Z.; Kasap, S.; Ertunc, S.; Kandemir, C. Evaluation of metabolic profiles of Saanen goats in the transition period. *J. Hell. Vet. Med. Soc.* **2020**, *71*, 2127–2134.
170. Sandabe, U.K.; Chaudhary, S.U.R. Effect of ambient temperature on some biochemical values in female Sahel goats. *Pak. Vet. J.* **2000**, *20*, 10–12. Available online: **https://www.pvj.com.pk/pdf-files/20_1/10-12.pdf** (accessed on 21 March 2025).
171. Di Trana, A.; Celi, P.; Claps, S.; Fedele, V.; Rubino, R. The effect of warm season and nutrition on oxidative status and metabolic profile in dairy goats during mid-lactation. *Anim. Sci.* **2006**, *82*, 717–722.
172. Al-Eissa, M.S.; Alkahtani, S.; Al-Farraj, S.A.; Alarifi, S.A.; Al-Dahmash, B.; Al-Yahya, H. Seasonal variation effects on the composition of blood in Nubian ibex (Capra nubiana) in Saudi Arabia. *Afr. J. Biotechnol.* **2012**, *11*, 1283–1286.
173. Celi, P.; Di Trana, A.; Quaranta, A. Metabolic profile and oxidative status in goats during the peripartum period. *Aust. J. Exp. Agric.* **2008**, *48*, 1004–1008.
174. Antunović, Z.; Marić, I.; Klir, Ž.; Šerić, V.; Mioč, B.; Novoselec, J. Hematobiochemical profile and acid-base status of Croatian spotted goats of different ages. *Arch. Anim. Breed.* **2019**, *62*, 455–463.

175. Banerjee, D.; Upadhyay, R.C.; Chaudhary, U.B.; Kumar, R.; Singh, S.; De Ashutosh, S. Seasonal variations in physio-biochemical profiles of Indian goats in the paradigm of hot and cold climate. *Biol. Rhythm Res.* **2014**, *46*, 221–236.

176. Martínez-Grimaldo, R.E.; Quiroz-Rocha, G.F.; Domínguez, Y. Determination of reference limits for hematological analytes in adult dairy goats in the Mexican Altiplano. *J. Fac. Vet. Med. Anim. Husb.* **2018**, *65*, 121–129.

177. Mazzuca Pizetti, A.J.; Sarmiento, R.O.; Pintos, L.A.; Trova, G.B.; Binda, J.A.; Sánchez Negrette, O. Hematological and protein profile of rodeo goats in extensive productions from different regions of the province of Salta, Argentina. *J. Appl. Anim. Res.* **2021**, *49*, 239–246.

178. Arfuso, F.; Fazio, F.; Rizzo, M.; Marafioti, S.; Zanghì, E.; Piccione, G. Factors affecting the hematological parameters in different goat breeds from Italy. *Ann. Anim. Sci.* **2016**, *16*, 743–757.

179. Tibbo, M.; Jibril, Y.; Woldemeskel, M.; Dawo, F.; Aragaw, K.; Rege, J.E.O. Factors affecting hematological profiles in three indigenous goat breeds from Ethiopia. *Int. J. Appl. Res. Vet. Med.* **2004**, *2*, 297–309. Available online: **https://www.cabidigitallibrary.org/doi/full/10.5555/20053025070** (a ccessed on 21 March 2025).

180. Piccione, G.; Monteverde, V.; Rizzo, M.; Vazzana, I.; Assenza, A.; Zumbo, A.; Niutta, P.P. Reference intervals of some electrophoretic and hematological parameters in Italian goats: Comparison between Girgentana and Aspromontana breeds. *J. Appl. Anim. Res.* **2014**, *42*, 434–439.

181. Al-Bulushi, S.; Shawaf, T.; Al-Hasani, A. Some hematological and biochemical parameters of different goat breeds in the Sultanate of Oman: A preliminary study. *Vet. World* **2017**, *10*, 461–466.

182. Abdalla, A.M.; Ibrahim, M.Y.; Hassan, Y.Y. Seasonal variation of red blood cell and leukocyte indices and serum proteins in female Nubian goats. *Middle-East J. Sci. Res.* **2009**, *4*, 168–174. Available online: **https://www.researchgate.net/profile/Abdalla-Abdelatif-2/publication/242210780_Seasonal_Variation_in_Erythrocytic_and_Leukocytic_Indices_and_Serum_Proteins_of_Female_Nubian_Goats/links/56c5c6cc08ae736e70491ffd/Seasonal-Variation-in-Erythrocytic-and-Leukocytic-Indices-and-Serum-Proteins-of-Female-Nubian-Goats.pdf** (accessed on 22 March 2025).

183. Bezerra, L.R.; Ferreira, A.F.; Camboim, E.K.A.; Justiniano, S.V.; Machado, P.C.R.; Gomes, B.B. Hematological profile of clinically sad goats raised in Cariri Paraíba. *Ciênc. Agrotec.* **2008**, *32*, 955–960.

184. Habibu, B.; Kawu, M.U.; Makun, H.J.; Aluwong, T.; Yaqub, L.S.; Ahmad, M.S.; Tauheed, M.; Buhari, H.U. Influence of sex, reproductive status and number of fetuses on erythrocyte osmotic fragility, hematological and physiological parameters in goats during hot and dry season. *Vet. Med.* **2014**, *59*, 479–490.

185. Agradi, S.; Menchetti, L.; Curone, G.; Faustini, M.; Vigo, D.; Villa, L.; Zanzani, S.A.; Postoli, R.; Kika, T.S.; Riva, F.; et al. Comparison of hematological parameters of Verzaschese and Camosciata delle Alpi goat dams in the context of adaptation to local environmental conditions in semi-extensive systems in Italy. *Animals* **2022**, *12*, 1703.

186. Silva, E.M.N.; de Souza, B.B.; de Assis Silva, G.; Cézar, M.F.; Soares Freitas, M.M.; Alves Benicio, T.M. Hematological evaluation of exotic and native goats in the semi-arid Paraíba region. *Ciênc. Agrotec.* **2008**, *32*, 561–566.

187. Hernández Martínez, B.; Murillo Ortiz, M.; Pámanes Carrasco, G.; Reyes Estrada, O.; Herrera Torres, E. Parámetros de fermentación y cinética ruminal en novillos suplementados con diferentes aditivos. *Investig. Cienc.* **2017**, *25*, 5–11. Available online: **https://www.redalyc.org/journal/674/67453654001/html/** (accessed on 22 March 2025).
188. Dhuha, J.M.; Muayad, M.T.A.; Saeed, O.A.; Al-Bayar, M.A.; Saeid, Z.J.M.; Al Bakri, S.A.; Che Musa, H.; Safaa, A.; Abed, Q.N.; Kaabi, S.A.G.; et al. Tropical seasonal changes impact on hematological parameters of goats. *J. Indones. Trop. Anim. Agric.* **2021**, *46*, 219–226.
189. Osman, I.N.E.H.; Al-Busaidi, R.M.; Johnson, E.H. Effects of age, breed and sex on hematological parameters of growing Omani goat breeds. *Sultan Qaboos Univ. J. Sci.* **2016**, *21*, 82–88.
190. Habibu, B.; Kawu, M.U.; Aluwong, T.; Makun, H.J. Influence of seasonal changes on physiological, hematological and serum thyroid hormone profile variables in male goats of the Red Sokoto and Sahel breeds. *J. Appl. Anim. Res.* **2017**, *45*, 55–64.
191. Azab, M.E.; Abdel-Maksoud, H.A. Changes in some hematological and biochemical parameters during prepartum and postpartum periods in female Baladi goats. *Small Rumin. Res.* **1999**, *34*, 77–85.
192. Roberto, J.V.B.; de Souza, B.B.; Da Silva, A.L.N.; Justiniano, S.V.; Soares Freitas, M.M. Hematological parameters of cutting goats subjected to different levels of supplementation in the semi-arid Paraíba region. *Caatinga Mag.* **2010**, *23*, 127–132. Available online: **https://www.redalyc.org/pdf/2371/237117582019.pdf** (accessed on 22 March 2025).

193. Walkden-Brown, S.W.; Norton, B.W.; Restall, B.J. Seasonal variation in voluntary feed intake and growth in cashmere males fed ad libitum on low- or high-quality diets. *Aust. J. Agric. Res.* **1994**, *45*, 355–366.

194. Alaku, O.; Moruppa, S.M. Dry-season weight loss in Red Sokoto (Maradi) goats reared in the Sahel region of northeastern Nigeria. *Int. J. Biometeorol.* **1983**, *27*, 143–156.

195. Souri, M.; Mirmahmoudi, R. Effect of season on dry matter intake and reproductive performance of Merghoz bucks in western Iran. *Iran. J. Appl. Anim. Sci.* **2014**, *4*, 317. Available online: **https://openurl.ebsco.com/EPDB%3Agcd%3A9%3A33086745/detailv2?sid=ebsco%3Aplink%3Ascholar&id=ebsco%3Agcd%3A113893608&crl=c&link_origin=scholar.google.com.ec** (accessed on 22 March 2025).

196. Hary, I.; Schwartz, H.-J. Effects of seasonal breeding on the productive performance of pastoral goat herds in northern Kenya: A longitudinal analysis of offspring growth and body weight development in goats. *J. Arid Environ.* **2002**, *50*, 641–664.

197. Yue, B.; Luo, X.; Yu, Z.; Mani, S.; Wang, Z.; Dou, W. Inflammatory Bowel Disease: A Potential Result from the Collusion between Gut Microbiota and Mucosal Immune System. *Microorganisms* **2019**, *7*, 440.

198. Zhao, M.; Burisch, J. Impact of Genes and the Environment on the Pathogenesis and Disease Course of Inflammatory Bowel Disease. *Dig. Dis. Sci.* **2019**, *64*, 1759–1769.

199. Baydi, Z.; Limami, Y.; Khalki, L.; Zaid, N.; Naya, A.; Mtairag, E.M.; Oudghiri, M.; Zaid, Y. An Update of Research Animal Models of Inflammatory Bowel Disease. *Sci. World J.* **2021**, *2021*, 7479540

200. Preksha, G.; Yesheswini, R.; Srikanth, C.V. Cell culture techniques in gastrointestinal research: Methods, possibilities and challenges. *Indian J. Pathol. Microbiol.* **2021**, *64* (Suppl. S1), S52–S57.
201. d'Aldebert, E.; Quaranta, M.; Sébert, M.; Bonnet, D.; Kirzin, S.; Portier, G.; Duffas, J.P.; Chabot, S.; Lluel, P.; Allart, S.; et al. Characterization of Human Colon Organoids From Inflammatory Bowel Disease Patients. *Front. Cell Dev. Biol.* **2020**, *8*, 363.
202. Xian, C.; Zhang, J.; Zhao, S.; Li, X.G. Gut-on-a-chip for disease models. *J. Tissue Eng.* **2023**, *14*, 20417314221149882.
203. Barker, N.; Huch, M.; Kujala, P.; van de Wetering, M.; Snippert, H.J.; van Es, J.H.; Sato, T.; Stange, D.E.; Begthel, H.; van den Born, M.; et al. Lgr5(+ve) stem cells drive self-renewal in the stomach and build long-lived gastric units in vitro. *Cell Stem Cell* **2010**, *6*, 25–36.
204. Barker, N.; van Es, J.H.; Kuipers, J.; Kujala, P.; van den Born, M.; Cozijnsen, M.; Haegebarth, A.; Korving, J.; Begthel, H.; Peters, P.J.; et al. Identification of stem cells in small intestine and colon by marker gene Lgr5. *Nature* **2007**, *449*, 1003–1007.
205. Sato, T.; Vries, R.G.; Snippert, H.J.; van de Wetering, M.; Barker, N.; Stange, D.E.; van Es, J.H.; Abo, A.; Kujala, P.; Peters, P.J.; et al. Single Lgr5 stem cells build crypt-villus structures in vitro without a mesenchymal niche. *Nature* **2009**, *459*, 262–265.
206. Xiao, S.; Zhou, L. Gastric Stem Cells: Physiological and Pathological Perspectives. *Front. Cell Dev. Biol.* **2020**, *8*, 571536.
207. Vivarelli, S.; Candido, S.; Caruso, G.; Falzone, L.; Libra, M. Patient-Derived Tumor Organoids for Drug Repositioning in Cancer Care: A Promising Approach in the Era of Tailored Treatment. *Cancers* **2020**, *12*, 3636.

208. Kim, J.; Koo, B.K.; Knoblich, J.A. Human organoids: Model systems for human biology and medicine. *Nat. Rev. Mol. Cell Biol.* **2020**, *21*, 571–584.
209. Singh, A.; Yadav, C.B.; Tabassum, N.; Bajpeyee, A.K.; Verma, V. Stem cell niche: Dynamic neighbor of stem cells. *Eur. J. Cell Biol.* **2019**, *98*, 65–73.
210. Lin, G.; Zhang, X.; Ren, J.; Pang, Z.; Wang, C.; Xu, N.; Xi, R. Integrin signaling is required for maintenance and proliferation of intestinal stem cells in Drosophila. *Dev. Biol.* **2013**, *377*, 177–187.
211. Schutgens, F.; Verhaar, M.C.; Rookmaaker, M.B. Pluripotent stem cell-derived kidney organoids: An in vivo-like in vitro technology. *Eur. J. Pharmacol.* **2016**, *790*, 12–20.
212. Hamilton, C.A.; Young, R.; Jayaraman, S.; Sehgal, A.; Paxton, E.; Thomson, S.; Katzer, F.; Hope, J.; Innes, E.; Morrison, L.J.; et al. Development of in vitro enteroids derived from bovine small intestinal crypts. *Vet. Res.* **2018**, *49*, 54.
213. Yang, B.; Fu, L.; Privratsky, J.R.; Lu, X.; Ren, J.; Mei, C.; Crowley, S.D. Interleukin-1 receptor activation aggravates autosomal dominant polycystic kidney disease by modulating regulated necrosis. *Am. J. Physiol. Renal Physiol.* **2019**, *317*, F221–F228.
214. Dinarello, C.A. Biologic basis for interleukin-1 in disease. *Blood* **1996**, *87*, 2095–2147.
215. Takeuchi, O.; Akira, S. Pattern recognition receptors and inflammation. *Cell* **2010**, *140*, 805–820.
216. Al-Sadi, R.M.; Ma, T.Y. IL-1beta causes an increase in intestinal epithelial tight junction permeability. *J. Immunol.* **2007**, *178*, 4641–4649.
217. Smith, D.; Price, D.R.G.; Burrells, A.; Faber, M.N.; Hildersley, K.A.; Chintoan-Uta, C.; Chapuis, A.F.; Stevens, M.; Stevenson, K.; Burgess,

S.T.G.; et al. The Development of Ovine Gastric and Intestinal Organoids for Studying Ruminant Host-Pathogen Interactions. *Front. Cell. Infect. Microbiol.* **2021**, *11*, 733811.

218. Fujii, M.; Matano, M.; Toshimitsu, K.; Takano, A.; Mikami, Y.; Nishikori, S.; Sugimoto, S.; Sato, T. Human Intestinal Organoids Maintain Self-Renewal Capacity and Cellular Diversity in Niche-Inspired Culture Condition. *Cell Stem Cell* **2018**, *23*, 787–793.e786.
219. Juul, A.; Bang, P.; Hertel, N.T.; Main, K.; Dalgaard, P.; Jørgensen, K.; Müller, J.; Hall, K.; Skakkebaek, N.E. Serum insulin-like growth factor-I in 1030 healthy children, adolescents, and adults: Relation to age, sex, stage of puberty, testicular size, and body mass index. *J. Clin. Endocrinol. Metab.* **1994**, *78*, 744–752.
220. Mah, A.T.; Van Landeghem, L.; Gavin, H.E.; Magness, S.T.; Lund, P.K. Impact of diet-induced obesity on intestinal stem cells: Hyperproliferation but impaired intrinsic function that requires insulin/IGF1. *Endocrinology* **2014**, *155*, 3302–3314.
221. Song, X.; Dai, D.; He, X.; Zhu, S.; Yao, Y.; Gao, H.; Wang, J.; Qu, F.; Qiu, J.; Wang, H.; et al. Growth Factor FGF2 Cooperates with Interleukin-17 to Repair Intestinal Epithelial Damage. *Immunity* **2015**, *43*, 488–501.
222. Di Giorgio, C.; Roselli, R.; Biagioli, M.; Bordoni, M.; Ricci, P.; Zampella, A.; Distrutti, E.; Donini, A.; Fiorucci, S. Modeling Inflammatory Bowel Disease by Intestinal Organoids. *Recent Adv. Inflamm. Allergy Drug Discov.* **2023**, *17*, 39–53.
223. Dotti, I.; Mayorgas, A.; Salas, A. Generation of human colon organoids from healthy and inflammatory bowel disease mucosa. *PLoS ONE* **2022**, *17*, e0276195.

224. Foley, K.E. Organoids: A better in vitro model. *Nat. Methods* **2017**, *14*, 559–562.
225. Blangy-Letheule, A.; Vergnaud, A.; Dupas, T.; Rozec, B.; Lauzier, B.; Leroux, A.A. Spontaneous Sepsis in Adult Horses: From Veterinary to Human Medicine Perspectives. *Cells* **2023**, *12*, 1052.
226. Lewis, D.H.; Chan, D.L.; Pinheiro, D.; Armitage-Chan, E.; Garden, O.A. The immunopathology of sepsis: Pathogen recognition, systemic inflammation, the compensatory anti-inflammatory response, and regulatory T cells. *J. Vet. Intern. Med.* **2012**, *26*, 457–482.
227. Prest, J.; Nguyen, T.; Rajah, T.; Prest, A.B.; Sathananthan, M.; Jeganathan, N. Sepsis-Related Mortality Rates and Trends Based on Site of Infection. *Crit. Care Explor.* **2022**, *4*, e0775.
228. Fleischmann, C.; Reichert, F.; Cassini, A.; Horner, R.; Harder, T.; Markwart, R.; Tröndle, M.; Savova, Y.; Kissoon, N.; Schlattmann, P.; et al. Global incidence and mortality of neonatal sepsis: A systematic review and meta-analysis. *Arch. Dis. Child.* **2021**, *106*, 745–752.
229. Taylor, S. A review of equine sepsis. *Equine Vet. Educ.* **2015**, *27*, 99–109. Sheats, M.K. A Comparative Review of Equine SIRS, Sepsis, and Neutrophils. *Front. Vet. Sci.* **2019**, *6*, 69.
230. Singer, M.; Deutschman, C.S.; Seymour, C.W.; Shankar-Hari, M.; Annane, D.; Bauer, M.; Bellomo, R.; Bernard, G.R.; Chiche, J.-D.; Coopersmith, C.M.; et al. The Third International Consensus Definitions for Sepsis and Septic Shock (Sepsis-3). *JAMA* **2016**, *315*, 801–810.
231. American College of Chest Physicians/Society of Critical Care Medicine Consensus Conference: Definitions for sepsis and organ failure and guidelines

for the use of innovative therapies in sepsis. *Crit. Care Med.* **1992**, *20*, 864–874.

232. Roy, M.F.; Kwong, G.P.; Lambert, J.; Massie, S.; Lockhart, S. Prognostic Value and Development of a Scoring System in Horses With Systemic Inflammatory Response Syndrome. *J. Vet. Intern. Med.* **2017**, *31*, 582–592.
233. Hotchkiss, R.S.; Monneret, G.; Payen, D. Sepsis-induced immunosuppression: From cellular dysfunctions to immunotherapy. *Nat. Rev. Immunol.* **2013**, *13*, 862–874.
234. Schulte, W.; Bernhagen, J.; Bucala, R. Cytokines in sepsis: Potent immunoregulators and potential therapeutic targets—An updated view. *Mediators Inflamm.* **2013**, *2013*, 165974.
235. Cao, C.; Yu, M.; Chai, Y. Pathological alteration and therapeutic implications of sepsis-induced immune cell apoptosis. *Cell Death Dis.* **2019**, *10*, 782.
236. Liu, C.; Chu, D.; Kalantar-Zadeh, K.; George, J.; Young, H.A.; Liu, G. Cytokines: From Clinical Significance to Quantification. *Adv. Sci.* **2021**, *8*, e2004433.
237. Zhang, H.; Wang, Y.; Qu, M.; Li, W.; Wu, D.; Cata, J.P.; Miao, C. Neutrophil, neutrophil extracellular traps and endothelial cell dysfunction in sepsis. *Clin. Transl. Med.* **2023**, *13*, e1170.
238. Gårdlund, B.; Sjölin, J.; Nilsson, A.; Roll, M.; Wickerts, C.J.; Wretlind, B. Plasma levels of cytokines in primary septic shock in humans: Correlation with disease severity. *J. Infect. Dis.* **1995**, *172*, 296–301.
239. Gharamti, A.; Samara, O.; Monzon, A.; Scherger, S.; DeSanto, K.; Sillau, S.; Franco-Paredes, C.; Henao-Martínez, A.; Shapiro, L. Association between cytokine levels, sepsis severity and clinical outcomes in sepsis: A quantitative systematic review protocol. *BMJ Open* **2021**, *11*, e048476.

240. Zhang, J.M.; An, J. Cytokines, inflammation, and pain. *Int. Anesthesiol. Clin.* **2007**, *45*, 27–37.
241. Wang, H.; Ma, S. The cytokine storm and factors determining the sequence and severity of organ dysfunction in multiple organ dysfunction syndrome. *Am. J. Emerg. Med.* **2008**, *26*, 711–715.
242. Arango Duque, G.; Descoteaux, A. Macrophage cytokines: Involvement in immunity and infectious diseases. *Front. Immunol.* **2014**, *5*, 491.
243. Dinarello, C.A. Historical insights into cytokines. *Eur. J. Immunol.* **2007**, *37* (Suppl. 1), S34–S45.
244. Tanaka, T.; Narazaki, M.; Kishimoto, T. IL-6 in inflammation, immunity, and disease. *Cold Spring Harb. Perspect. Biol.* **2014**, *6*, a016295.
245. Ludwig, E.K.; Hobbs, K.J.; McKinney-Aguirre, C.A.; Gonzalez, L.M. Biomarkers of Intestinal Injury in Colic. *Animals* **2023**, *13*, 227.
246. Xing, Z.; Gauldie, J.; Cox, G.; Baumann, H.; Jordana, M.; Lei, X.F.; Achong, M.K. IL-6 is an antiinflammatory cytokine required for controlling local or systemic acute inflammatory responses. *J. Clin. Investig.* **1998**, *101*, 311–320.
247. Molano Franco, D.; Arevalo-Rodriguez, I.; Roqué, I.F.M.; Montero Oleas, N.G.; Nuvials, X.; Zamora, J. Plasma interleukin-6 concentration for the diagnosis of sepsis in critically ill adults. *Cochrane Database Syst. Rev.* **2019**, *4*, Cd011811.
248. Vivas, M.C.; Villamarin Guerrero, H.F.; Tascon, A.J.; Valderrama-Aguirre, A. Plasma interleukin-6 levels correlate with survival in patients with bacterial sepsis and septic shock. *Interv. Med. Appl. Sci.* **2021**, *11*, 224–230.
249. Morris, D.D.; Moore, J.N.; Crowe, N.; Moldawer, L.L. Effect of experimentally induced endotoxemia on serum interleukin-6 activity in horses. *Am. J. Vet. Res.* **1992**, *53*, 753–756.

250. Barton, M.H.; Collatos, C. Tumor necrosis factor and interleukin-6 activity and endotoxin concentration in peritoneal fluid and blood of horses with acute abdominal disease. *J. Vet. Intern. Med.* **1999**, *13*, 457–464
251. Fedorka, C.E.; Scoggin, K.E.; Ali, H.E.; Loux, S.C.; Dini, P.; Troedsson, M.H.T.; Ball, B.A. Interleukin-6 pathobiology in equine placental infection. *Am. J. Reprod. Immunol.* **2021**, *85*, e13363
252. Zak, A.; Siwinska, N.; Elzinga, S.; Barker, V.; Stefaniak, T.; Schanbacher, B.; Place, N.; Niedzwiedz, A.; Adams, A. Effects of equine metabolic syndrome on inflammation and acute-phase markers in horses. *Domest. Anim. Endocrinol.* **2020**, *72*, 106448.
253. Guo, H.-L.; Shi, F.-D.; Zhou, Q.; Liu, Q.-Y.; Wang, Y.-X.; Song, Y.; Wu, Z.-S.; Shi, Y.-H.; Zhang, L.; Xu, K.-Z.; et al. Interleukin-1β Protection Against Experimental Sepsis in Mice. *Inflammation* **2021**, *44*, 358–370.
254. Lemon, J.K.; Miller, M.R.; Weiser, J.N. Sensing of interleukin-1 cytokines during Streptococcus pneumoniae colonization contributes to macrophage recruitment and bacterial clearance. *Infect. Immun.* **2015**, *83*, 3204–3212.
255. Jiménez-Sousa, M.; Medrano, L.M.; Liu, P.; Almansa, R.; Fernández-Rodríguez, A.; Gómez-Sánchez, E.; Rico, L.; Heredia-Rodríguez, M.; Gómez-Pesquera, E.; Tamayo, E.; et al. IL-1B rs16944 polymorphism is related to septic shock and death. *Eur. J. Clin. Investig.* **2017**, *47*, 53–62.
256. Wen, A.Q.; Gu, W.; Wang, J.; Feng, K.; Qin, L.; Ying, C.; Zhu, P.F.; Wang, Z.G.; Jiang, J.X. Clinical relevance of IL-1beta promoter polymorphisms (-1470, -511, and -31) in patients with major trauma. *Shock* **2010**, *33*, 576–582.
257. Tadros, E.M.; Frank, N. Effects of continuous or intermittent lipopolysaccharide administration for 48 hours on the systemic inflammatory response in horses. *Am. J. Vet. Res.* **2012**, *73*, 1394–1402.

258. Castagnetti, C.; Mariella, J.; Pirrone, A.; Cinotti, S.; Mari, G.; Peli, A. Expression of interleukin-1β, interleukin-8, and interferon-γ in blood samples obtained from healthy and sick neonatal foals. *Am. J. Vet. Res.* **2012**, *73*, 1418–1427.
259. Jang, D.-I.; Lee, A.-H.; Shin, H.-Y.; Song, H.-R.; Park, J.-H.; Kang, T.-B.; Lee, S.-R.; Yang, S.-H. The Role of Tumor Necrosis Factor Alpha (TNF-α) in Autoimmune Disease and Current TNF-α Inhibitors in Therapeutics. *Int. J. Mol. Sci.* **2021**, *22*, 2719.
260. Spooner, C.E.; Markowitz, N.P.; Saravolatz, L.D. The role of tumor necrosis factor in sepsis. *Clin. Immunol. Immunopathol.* **1992**, *62 Pt 2*, S11–S17.
261. Gharamti, A.A.; Samara, O.; Monzon, A.; Montalbano, G.; Scherger, S.; DeSanto, K.; Chastain, D.B.; Sillau, S.; Montoya, J.G.; Franco-Paredes, C.; et al. Proinflammatory cytokines levels in sepsis and healthy volunteers, and tumor necrosis factor-alpha associated sepsis mortality: A systematic review and meta-analysis. *Cytokine* **2022**, *158*, 156006.
262. Rigato, O.; Ujvari, S.; Castelo, A.; Salomão, R. Tumor necrosis factor alpha (TNF-α) and sepsis: Evidence for a role in host defense. *Infection* **1996**, *24*,
263. Menzies-Gow, N.J.; Wray, H.; Bailey, S.R.; Harris, P.A.; Elliott, J. The effect of tumour necrosis factor-α and insulin on equine digital blood vessel function in vitro. *Inflamm. Res.* **2014**, *63*, 637–647.
264. Aamer, H.G.; El-Ashker, M.R.; Nour, E.M.; Wafa, E.W.; Youssef, M.A. Sepsis-Induced Acute Kidney Injury in Equine: Current Knowledge and Future Perspectives. *J. Equine Vet. Sci.* **2017**, *50*, 84–95.
265. Morris, D.D.; Moore, J.N.; Crowe, N. Serum tumor necrosis factor activity in horses with colic attributable to gastrointestinal tract disease. *Am. J. Vet. Res.* **1991**, *52*, 1565–1569.

266. Bergmann, C.B.; Beckmann, N.; Salyer, C.E.; Hanschen, M.; Crisologo, P.A.; Caldwell, C.C. Potential Targets to Mitigate Trauma- or Sepsis-Induced Immune Suppression. *Front. Immunol.* **2021**, *12*, 622601
267. Dang, P.M.; Elbim, C.; Marie, J.C.; Chiandotto, M.; Gougerot-Pocidalo, M.A.; El-Benna, J. Anti-inflammatory effect of interleukin-10 on human neutrophil respiratory burst involves inhibition of GM-CSF-induced p47PHOX phosphorylation through a decrease in ERK1/2 activity. *FASEB J.* **2006**, *20*, 1504–1506.
268. L'Heureux, M.; Kashiouris, M.; Fowler, A.; Fisher, B. ASSOCIATION BETWEEN IL-10 AND MORTALITY IN SEPSIS-INDUCED ARDS. *Chest* **2020**, *158* (Suppl. 4), A621.
269. Pusterla, N.; Magdesian, K.G.; Mapes, S.; Leutenegger, C.M. Expression of molecular markers in blood of neonatal foals with sepsis. *Am. J. Vet. Res.* **2006**, *67*, 1045–1049.
270. Karbian, N.; Abutbul, A.; El-Amore, R.; Eliaz, R.; Beeri, R.; Reicher, B.; Mevorach, D. Apoptotic cell therapy for cytokine storm associated with acute severe sepsis. *Cell Death Dis.* **2020**, *11*, 535.
271. Hernandez, A.V.; Piscoya, A.; Pasupuleti, V.; Phan, M.T.; Julakanti, S.; Khen, P.; Roman, Y.M.; Carranza-Tamayo, C.O.; Escobedo, A.A.; White, C.M. Beneficial and Harmful Effects of Monoclonal Antibodies for the Treatment and Prophylaxis of COVID-19: Systematic Review and Meta-Analysis. *Am. J. Med.* **2022**, *135*, 1349–1361.e18.
272. Acchione, M.; Kwon, H.; Jochheim, C.M.; Atkins, W.M. Impact of linker and conjugation chemistry on antigen binding, Fc receptor binding and thermal stability of model antibody-drug conjugates. *mAbs* **2012**, *4*, 362–372.

273. Cargile, J.L.; MacKay, R.J.; Dankert, J.R.; Skelley, L. Effect of treatment with a monoclonal antibody against equine tumor necrosis factor (TNF) on clinical, hematologic, and circulating TNF responses of miniature horses given endotoxin. *Am. J. Vet. Res.* **1995**, *56*, 1451–1459.
274. Cargile, J.L.; MacKay, R.J.; Dankert, J.R.; Skelley, L. Effects of tumor necrosis factor blockade on interleukin 6, lactate, thromboxane, and prostacyclin responses in miniature horses given endotoxin. *Am. J. Vet. Res.* **1995**, *56*, 1445–1450.
275. Langreder, N.; Schäckermann, D.; Meier, D.; Becker, M.; Schubert, M.; Dübel, S.; Reinard, T.; Figge-Wegener, S.; Roßbach, K.; Bäumer, W.; et al. Development of an inhibiting antibody against equine interleukin 5 to treat insect bite hypersensitivity of horses. *Sci. Rep.* **2023**, *13*, 4029.
276. Zahavi, D.; Weiner, L. Monoclonal Antibodies in Cancer Therapy. *Antibodies* **2020**, *9*, 34.
277. Hamilton, F.W.; Thomas, M.; Arnold, D.; Palmer, T.; Moran, E.; Mentzer, A.J.; Maskell, N.; Baillie, K.; Summers, C.; Hingorani, A.; et al. Therapeutic potential of IL6R blockade for the treatment of sepsis and sepsis-related death: A Mendelian randomisation study. *PLoS Med.* **2023**, *20*, e1004174.
278. Alsabani, M.; Abrams, S.T.; Cheng, Z.; Morton, B.; Lane, S.; Alosaimi, S.; Yu, W.; Wang, G.; Toh, C.H. Reduction of NETosis by targeting CXCR1/2 reduces thrombosis, lung injury, and mortality in experimental human and murine sepsis. *Br. J. Anaesth.* **2022**, *128*, 283–293.
279. Lasarzik, J.; Lischer, C.J.; Ehrle, A.; Estrada, R.; Rettig, M.; Klaus, C.; Einspanier, R.; Bondzio, A. Interleukin-1 Receptor Antagonist and Interleukin-1 Beta Levels in Equine Synovial Fluid of Normal and

Osteoarthritic Joints: Influence of Anatomic Joint Location and Repeated Arthrocentesis. *J. Equine Vet. Sci.* **2016**, *42*, 67–72.

280. Friesecke, S.; Stecher, S.S.; Gross, S.; Felix, S.B.; Nierhaus, A. Extracorporeal cytokine elimination as rescue therapy in refractory septic shock: A prospective single-center study. *J. Artif. Organs* **2017**, *20*, 252–259.
281. Terayama, T.; Yamakawa, K.; Umemura, Y.; Aihara, M.; Fujimi, S. Polymyxin B Hemoperfusion for Sepsis and Septic Shock: A Systematic Review and Meta-Analysis. *Surg. Infect.* **2017**, *18*, 225–233.
282. Gocho, T.; Mori, H.; Islam, M.; Maruchi, Y.; Takenaka, N.; Tomino, A.; Tsuda, M.; Kano, H.; Takeyama, N.; Islam, M. Removal of Circulating Neutrophil Extracellular Trap Components with an Immobilized Polymyxin B Filter: A Preliminary Study. *Shock* **2020**, *54*, 44–49.
283. Jansen, A.; Waalders, N.J.B.; van Lier, D.P.T.; Kox, M.; Pickkers, P. CytoSorb hemoperfusion markedly attenuates circulating cytokine concentrations during systemic inflammation in humans in vivo. *Crit. Care* **2023**, *27*, 117.
284. Träger, K.; Skrabal, C.; Fischer, G.; Schroeder, J.; Marenski, L.; Liebold, A.; Reinelt, H.; Datzmann, T. Hemoadsorption treatment with CytoSorb(®) in patients with extracorporeal life support therapy: A case series. *Int. J. Artif. Organs* **2020**, *43*, 422–429.
285. Li, W.; Chen, Y.; Li, D.; Meng, X.; Liu, Z.; Liu, Y.; Fan, H. Hemoadsorption in acute respiratory distress syndrome patients requiring venovenous extracorporeal membrane oxygenation: A systematic review. *Respir. Res.* **2024**, *25*, 27.
286. Anisimova, N.Y.; Gromova, E.G.; Kuznetsova, L.S.; Sitdikova, S.M.; Kiselevskii, M.V. Dynamics of elimination of bacterial endotoxins and

cytokines from the blood of tumor patients with sepsis in hemoperfusion using carbon adsorbents. *Bull. Exp. Biol. Med.* **2011**, *151*, 622–624.

287. Hobbs, K.; Davis, J.; Cooper, B.; Ueda, Y.; Burke, M.; Sheats, M. Hemadsorption extracorporeal therapy removes cytokines ex vivo in horses. *Am. J. Vet. Res.* **2024**, *85*, 1–8.
288. Hobbs, K.J.; Le Sueur, A.N.V.; Burke, M.J.; Cooper, B.L.; Sheats, M.K.; Ueda, Y. Feasibility of hemoperfusion using extracorporeal therapy in the horse. *Front. Vet. Sci.* **2024**, *11*, 1414426.
289. Hobbs, K.J.; Le Sueur, A.N.V.; Hallowell, K.; Martin, E.; Sheats, M.K.; Ueda, Y. Use of extracorporeal hemoperfusion therapy in an adult horse with *Clostridioides difficile* colitis and severe systemic inflammatory response syndrome. *J. Vet. Intern. Med.* **2024**.
290. Honore, P.M.; Hoste, E.; Molnár, Z.; Jacobs, R.; Joannes-Boyau, O.; Malbrain, M.; Forni, L.G. Cytokine removal in human septic shock: Where are we and where are we going? *Ann. Intensive Care* **2019**, *9*, 56.
291. Kanjo, A.; Molnar, Z.; Zádori, N.; Gede, N.; Erőss, B.; Szakó, L.; Kiss, T.; Márton, Z.; Malbrain, M.L.N.G.; Szuldrzynski, K.; et al. Dosing of Extracorporeal Cytokine Removal In Septic Shock (DECRISS): Protocol of a prospective, randomised, adaptive, multicentre clinical trial. *BMJ Open* **2021**, *11*, e050464.
292. Lisowski, Z.M.; Pirie, R.S.; Blikslager, A.T.; Lefebvre, D.; Hume, D.A.; Hudson, N.P.H. An update on equine post-operative ileus: Definitions, pathophysiology and management. *Equine Vet. J.* **2018**, *2*, 292–303.
293. Vather, R.; O'Grady, G.; Bissett, I.P.; Dinning, P.G. Postoperative ileus: Mechanisms and future directions for research. *Clin. Exp. Pharmacol. Physiol.* **2014**, *2*, 358–370.

294. Fukuda, H.; Tsuchida, D.; Koda, K.; Miyazaki, M.; Pappas, T.N.; Takahashi, T. Inhibition of sympathetic pathways restores postoperative ileus in the upper and lower gastrointestinal tract. *J. Gastroenterol. Hepatol.* **2007**, *2*, 1293–1299.
295. Hellstrom, E.A.; Ziegler, A.L.; Blikslager, A.T. Postoperative Ileus: Comparative Pathophysiology and Future Therapies. *Front. Vet. Sci.* **2021**, *8*, 714800.
296. Lefebvre, D.; Hudson, N.P.H.; Elce, Y.A.; Blikslager, A.; Divers, T.J.; Handel, I.G.; Tremaine, W.H.; Pirie, R.S. Clinical features and management of equine post operative ileus (POI): Survey of Diplomates of the American Colleges of Veterinary Internal Medicine (ACVIM), Veterinary Surgeons (ACVS) and Veterinary Emergency and Critical Care (ACVECC). *Equine Vet. J.* **2016**, *2*, 714–719.
297. Lefebvre, D.; Pirie, R.S.; Handel, I.G.; Tremaine, W.H.; Hudson, N.P. Clinical features and management of equine post operative ileus: Survey of diplomates of the European Colleges of Equine Internal Medicine (ECEIM) and Veterinary Surgeons (ECVS). *Equine Vet. J.* **2016**, *2*, 182–187.
298. Berghmans, T.M.; Hulsewé, K.W.; Buurman, W.A.; Luyer, M.D. Stimulation of the autonomic nervous system in colorectal surgery: A study protocol for a randomized controlled trial. *Trials* **2012**, *13*, 93.
299. Helman, C.A. Chewing gum is as effective as food in stimulating cephalic phase gastric secretion. *Am. J. Gastroenterol.* **1988**, *2*, 640–642. Giusto, G.; Pagliara, E.; Gandini, M. Effects of Bit Chewing on Right Upper Quadrant Intestinal Sound Frequency in Adult Horses. *J. Equine Vet. Sci.* **2014**, *2*, 520–523.

300. Butt, M.F.; Albusoda, A.; Farmer, A.D.; Aziz, Q. The anatomical basis for transcutaneous auricular vagus nerve stimulation. *J. Anat.* **2020**, *2*, 588–611.
301. He, W.; Wang, X.; Shi, H.; Shang, H.; Li, L.; Jing, X.; Zhu, B. Auricular acupuncture and vagal regulation. *Evid. Based Complement. Alternat Med.* **2012**, *2012*, 786839.
302. Asher, G.N.; Jonas, D.E.; Coeytaux, R.R.; Reilly, A.C.; Loh, Y.L.; Motsinger-Reif, A.A.; Winham, S.J. Auriculotherapy for pain management: A systematic review and meta-analysis of randomized controlled trials. *J. Altern. Complement. Med.* **2010**, *2*, 1097–1108.
303. Usichenko, T.; Hacker, H.; Lotze, M. Transcutaneous auricular vagal nerve stimulation (taVNS) might be a mechanism behind the analgesic effects of auricular acupuncture. *Brain Stimul.* **2017**, *2*, 1042–1044.
304. Ru, O.; Jin, X.; Qu, L.; Long, D.; Liu, M.; Cheng, L.; Jiang, Y. Low-intensity transcutaneous auricular vagus nerve stimulation reduces postoperative ileus after laparoscopic radical resection of colorectal cancer: A randomized controlled trial. *Minerva Anestesiol.* **2023**, *2*, 149–156.
305. Zhu, Y.; Xu, F.; Lu, D.; Rong, P.; Cheng, J.; Li, M.; Gong, Y.; Sun, C.; Wei, W.; Lin, L.; et al. Transcutaneous auricular vagal nerve stimulation improves functional dyspepsia by enhancing vagal efferent activity. *Am. J. Physiol. Gastrointest. Liver Physiol.* **2021**, *2*, G700–G711.
306. Vitale, V.; Balocchi, R.; Varanini, M.; Sgorbini, M.; Macerata, A.; Sighieri, C.; Baragli, P. The effects of restriction of movement on the reliability of heart rate variability measurements in the horse (*Equus caballus*). *J. Vet. Behavior.* **2013**, *2*, 400–403.

307. Tarvainen, M.P.; Niskanen, J.P.; Lipponen, J.A.; Ranta-Aho, P.O.; Karjalainen, P.A. Kubios HRV--heart rate variability analysis software. *Comput. Methods Programs Biomed.* **2014**, *2*, 210–220.
308. Mouchtouri, E.-T.; Lekkas, P.; Delis, F.; Pantelakis, E.; Mourouzis, I.; Pantos, C.; Kolettis, T.M. Sympathetic and Vagal Responses Elicited by Acute Stress in Rats. *Cureus* **2020**, *2*, e11602
309. Rietmann, T.; Stuart, A.; Bernasconi, P.; Stauffacher, M.; Auer, J.A.; Weishaupt, M.A. Assessment of mental stress in warmblood horses: Heart rate variability in comparison to heart rate and selected behavioural parameters. *Appl. Anim. Behav. Sci.* **2004**, *88*, 121–136.
310. Tekdemir, I.; Aslan, A.; Elhan, A. A clinico-anatomic study of the auricular branch of the vagus nerve and Arnold‘s ear-cough reflex. *Surg. Radiol. Anat.* **1998**, *2*, 253–257.
311. Yu, L.; Scherlag, B.J.; Li, S.; Fan, Y.; Dyer, J.; Male, S.; Varma, V.; Sha, Y.; Stavrakis, S.; Po, S.S. Low-level transcutaneous electrical stimulation of the auricular branch of the vagus nerve: A noninvasive approach to treat the initial phase of atrial fibrillation. *Heart Rhythm.* **2013**, *2*, 428–435.
312. Vitale, V.; Viu, J.; Armengou, L.; Ríos, J.; Jose-Cunilleras, E. Prognostic value of measuring heart rate variability at the time of hospital admission in horses with colic. *Am. J. Vet. Res.* **2020**, *2*, 147–152.
313. Hong, G.-S.; Pintea, B.; Lingohr, P.; Coch, C.; Randau, T.; Schaefer, N.; Wehner, S.; Kalff, J.C.; Pantelis, D. Effect of transcutaneous vagus nerve stimulation on muscle activity in the gastrointestinal tract (transVaGa): A prospective clinical trial. *Int. J. Color. Dis.* **2019**, *2*, 417–422.
314. Badran, B.; Glusman, C.; Badran, A.; Austelle, C.; DeVries, W.; Borckhardt, J.; George, M. The physiological and neurobiological effects of

transcutaneous auricular vagus nerve stimulation (taVNS). *Brain Stimul.* **2017**, *2*, 378.

315. Clancy, J.A.; Mary, D.A.; Witte, K.K.; Greenwood, J.P.; Deuchars, S.A.; Deuchars, J. Non-invasive vagus nerve stimulation in healthy humans reduces sympathetic nerve activity. *Brain Stimul.* **2014**, *2*, 871–877.
316. Groves, D.A.; Brown, V.J. Vagal nerve stimulation: A review of its applications and potential mechanisms that mediate its clinical effects. *Neurosci. Biobehav. Rev.* **2005**, *2*, 493–500.
317. Castoro, M.A.; Yoo, P.B.; Hincapie, J.G.; Hamann, J.J.; Ruble, S.B.; Wolf, P.D.; Grill, W.M. Excitation properties of the right cervical vagus nerve in adult dogs. *Exp. Neurol.* **2011**, *2*, 62–68.
318. Sluka, K.A.; Walsh, D. Transcutaneous electrical nerve stimulation: Basic science mechanisms and clinical effectiveness. *J. Pain.* **2003**, *2*, 109–121.
319. Safi, S.; Ellrich, J.; Neuhuber, W. Myelinated Axons in the Auricular Branch of the Human Vagus Nerve. *Anat. Rec.* **2016**, *2*, 1184–1191.
320. Thor, P.J.; Furgała, A.; Mazur, M.; Pośnik-Urbańska, A.; Kolasińska-Kloch, W.; Czarnecka, D.; Kawecka-Jaszcz, K. Comparison of cardiac and gastric responses to vagal stimulation in hypertensive women. *Med. Sci. Monit.* **2009**, *2*, Cr504–Cr511.
321. Sanders, K.M.; Ward, S.M. Interstitial cells of Cajal: A new perspective on smooth muscle function. *J. Physiol.* **2006**, *576 Pt 3*, 721–726.
322. Tracey, K.J. The inflammatory reflex. *Nature* **2002**, *2*, 853–859.
323. Broome, B.A. The impact of urinary incontinence on self-efficacy and quality of life. *Health Qual. Life Outcomes* **2003**, *1*, 35.
324. Fultz, N.H.; Herzog, A.R. Self-reported social and emotional impact of urinary incontinence. *J. Am. Geriatr. Soc.* **2001**, *49*, 892–899.

325. Subak, L.L.; Brubaker, L.; Chai, T.C.; Creasman, J.M.; Diokno, A.C.; Goode, P.S.; Kraus, S.R.; Kusek, J.W.; Leng, W.W.; Lukacz, E.S.; et al. High costs of urinary incontinence among women electing surgery to treat stress incontinence. *Obstet. Gynecol.* **2008**, *111*, 899–907.

326. Delancey, J.O. Why do women have stress urinary incontinence? *Neurourol. Urodyn.* **2010**, *29* (Suppl. S1), S13–S17

327. Markland, A.D.; Goode, P.S.; Redden, D.T.; Borrud, L.G.; Burgio, K.L. Prevalence of urinary incontinence in men: Results from the national health and nutrition examination survey. *J. Urol.* **2010**, *184*, 1022–1027.

328. Ptak, M.; Brodowska, A.; Ciećwież, S.; Rotter, I. Quality of Life in Women with Stage 1 Stress Urinary Incontinence after Application of Conservative Treatment—A Randomized Trial. *Int. J. Environ. Res. Public Health* **2017**, *14*, 577.

329. Hillary, C.J.; Roman, S.; MacNeil, S.; Aicher, W.K.; Stenzl, A.; Chapple, C.R. Regenerative medicine and injection therapies in stress urinary incontinence. *Nat. Rev. Urol.* **2020**, *17*, 151–161.

330. Harland, N.; Walz, S.; Eberli, D.; Schmid, F.A.; Aicher, W.K.; Stenzl, A.; Amend, B. Stress Urinary Incontinence: An Unsolved Clinical Challenge. *Biomedicines* **2023**, *11*, 2486.

331. Aicher, W.K.; Hart, M.L.; Stallkamp, J.; Klunder, M.; Ederer, M.; Sawodny, O.; Vaegler, M.; Amend, B.; Sievert, K.D.; Stenzl, A. Towards a Treatment of Stress Urinary Incontinence: Application of Mesenchymal Stromal Cells for Regeneration of the Sphincter Muscle. *J. Clin. Med.* **2014**, *3*, 197–215.

332. Schmid, F.A.; Williams, J.K.; Kessler, T.M.; Stenzl, A.; Aicher, W.K.; Andersson, K.E.; Eberli, D. Treatment of Stress Urinary Incontinence with

Muscle Stem Cells and Stem Cell Components: Chances, Challenges and Future Prospects. *Int. J. Mol. Sci.* **2021**, *22*, 3981.

333. Peters, K.M.; Dmochowski, R.R.; Carr, L.K.; Robert, M.; Kaufman, M.R.; Sirls, L.T.; Herschorn, S.; Birch, C.; Kultgen, P.L.; Chancellor, M.B. Autologous Muscle Derived Cells for Treatment of Stress Urinary Incontinence in Women. *J. Urol.* **2014**, *192*, 469–476.
334. Pokrywczynska, M.; Adamowicz, J.; Czapiewska, M.; Balcerczyk, D.; Jundzill, A.; Nowacki, M.; Petros, P.; Drewa, T. Targeted therapy for stress urinary incontinence: A systematic review based on clinical trials. *Expert. Opin. Biol. Ther.* **2016**, *16*, 233–242.
335. Vilsbøll, A.W.; Mouritsen, J.M.; Jensen, L.P.; Bødker, N.; Holst, A.W.; Pennisi, C.P.; Ehlers, L. Cell-based therapy for the treatment of female stress urinary incontinence: An early cost–effectiveness analysis. *Regen. Med.* **2018**, *13*, 321–330.
336. Alarcin, E.; Bal-Öztürk, A.; Avci, H.; Ghorbanpoor, H.; Dogan Guzel, F.; Akpek, A.; Yesiltas, G.; Canak-Ipek, T.; Avci-Adali, M. Current Strategies for the Regeneration of Skeletal Muscle Tissue. *Int. J. Mol. Sci.* **2021**, *22*, 5929.
337. Fang, J.; Sia, J.; Soto, J.; Wang, P.; Li, L.K.; Hsueh, Y.-Y.; Sun, R.; Faull, K.F.; Tidball, J.G.; Li, S. Skeletal muscle regeneration via the chemical induction and expansion of myogenic stem cells in situ or in vitro. *Nat. Biomed. Eng.* **2021**, *5*, 864–879.
338. Kelp, A.; Albrecht, A.; Amend, B.; Klunder, M.; Rapp, P.; Sawodny, O.; Stenzl, A.; Aicher, W.K. Establishing and monitoring of urethral sphincter deficiency in a large animal model. *World J. Urol.* **2017**, *35*, 1977–1986.

339. Metzger, K.; Tuchscherer, A.; Palin, M.F.; Ponsuksili, S.; Kalbe, C. Establishment and validation of cell pools using primary muscle cells derived from satellite cells of pig skeletal muscle. *In Vitro Cell Dev. Biol. Anim.* **2020**, *56*, 193–199.
340. Ding, S.; Wang, F.; Liu, Y.; Li, S.; Zhou, G.; Hu, P. Characterization and isolation of highly purified porcine satellite cells. *Cell Death Discov.* **2017**, *3*, 17003.
341. Brun, J.; Lutz, K.A.; Neumayer, K.M.; Klein, G.; Seeger, T.; Uynuk-Ool, T.; Worgotter, K.; Schmid, S.; Kraushaar, U.; Guenther, E.; et al. Smooth Muscle-Like Cells Generated from Human Mesenchymal Stromal Cells Display Marker Gene Expression and Electrophysiological Competence Comparable to Bladder Smooth Muscle Cells. *PLoS ONE* **2015**, *10*, e0145153.
342. Rasmussen, R.; Morrison, T.; Herrmann, M.; Wittwer, C. Quantitative PCR by continuous fluorescence monitoring of a double strand dna specific binding dye. *Biochemica* **1998**, *2*, 8–11.
343. Kobayashi-Kinoshita, S.; Yamakoshi, Y.; Onuma, K.; Yamamoto, R.; Asada, Y. TGF-Î²1 autocrine signalling and enamel matrix components. *Sci. Rep.* **2016**, *6*, 33644.
344. Kalbe, C.; Mau, M.; Rehfeldt, C. Developmental changes and the impact of isoflavones on mRNA expression of IGF-I receptor, EGF receptor and related growth factors in porcine skeletal muscle cell cultures. *Growth Horm. IGF Res.* **2008**, *18*, 424–433.
345. Zhang, S.; Chen, X.; Huang, Z.; Chen, D.; Yu, B.; Chen, H.; Luo, J.; He, J.; Zheng, P.; Yu, J. Leucine promotes differentiation of porcine myoblasts

through the protein kinase B (Akt)/Forkhead box O1 signalling pathway. *Br. J. Nutr.* **2018**, *119*, 727–733.

346. Geng, R.; Knoll, J.; Harland, N.; Amend, B.; Enderle, M.D.; Linzenbold, W.; Abruzzese, T.; Kalbe, C.; Kemter, E.; Wolf, E.; et al. Replacing Needle Injection by a Novel Waterjet Technology Grants Improved Muscle Cell Delivery in Target Tissues. *Cell Transplant.* **2022**, *31*, 9636897221080943.
347. Maak, S.; Wicke, M.; Swalve, H.H. Analysis of gene expression in specific muscle of swine and turkey. *Arch. Tierz.* **2005**, *48*, 135–140.
348. Pilz, G.A.; Braun, J.; Ulrich, C.; Felka, T.; Warstat, K.; Ruh, M.; Schewe, B.; Abele, H.; Larbi, A.; Aicher, W.K. Human mesenchymal stromal cells express CD14 cross-reactive epitopes. *Cytom. A* **2011**, *79*, 635–645.
349. Robinson, J.P. *Current Protocols in Cytometry*; John Wiley and Sons, Inc.: New York, NY, USA, 1998.
350. Amend, B.; Kelp, A.; Vaegler, M.; Klunder, M.; Frajs, V.; Klein, G.; Sievert, K.D.; Sawodny, O.; Stenzl, A.; Aicher, W.K. Precise injection of human mesenchymal stromal cells in the urethral sphincter complex of Gottingen minipigs without unspecific bulking effects. *Neurourol. Urodyn.* **2017**, *36*, 1723–1733.
351. Beck, J.; Horikawa, I.; Harris, C. Cellular Senescence: Mechanisms, Morphology, and Mouse Models. *Vet. Pathol.* **2020**, *57*, 747–757.
352. Seale, P.; Sabourin, L.A.; Girgis-Gabardo, A.; Mansouri, A.; Gruss, P.; Rudnicki, M.A. Pax7 is required for the specification of myogenic satellite cells. *Cell* **2000**, *102*, 777–786.
353. Hernández-Hernández, J.M.; García-González, E.G.; Brun, C.E.; Rudnicki, M.A. The myogenic regulatory factors, determinants of muscle development, cell identity and regeneration. *Semin. Cell Dev. Biol.* **2017**, *72*, 10–18.

354. Sinanan, A.C.; Hunt, N.P.; Lewis, M.P. Human adult craniofacial muscle-derived cells: Neural-cell adhesion-molecule (NCAM; CD56)-expressing cells appear to contain multipotential stem cells. *Biotechnol Appl Biochem.* **2004**, *40*, 25–34.
355. Capkovic, K.L.; Stevenson, S.; Johnson, M.C.; Thelen, J.J.; Cornelison, D.D. Neural cell adhesion molecule (NCAM) marks adult myogenic cells committed to differentiation. *Exp. Cell Res.* **2008**, *314*, 1553–1565.
356. Pisani, D.F.; Clement, N.; Loubat, A.; Plaisant, M.; Sacconi, S.; Kurzenne, J.Y.; Desnuelle, C.; Dani, C.; Dechesne, C.A. Hierarchization of myogenic and adipogenic progenitors within human skeletal muscle. *Stem Cells* **2010**, *28*, 2182–2194.
357. Capetanaki, Y.; Milner, D.J.; Weitzer, G. Desmin in muscle formation and maintenance: Knockouts and consequences. *Cell Struct. Funct.* **1997**, *22*, 103–116.
358. Hnia, K.; Ramspacher, C.; Vermot, J.; Laporte, J. Desmin in muscle and associated diseases: Beyond the structural function. *Cell Tissue Res.* **2015**, *360*, 591–608.
359. Schmidt, M.; Schüler, S.C.; Hüttner, S.S.; von Eyss, B.; von Maltzahn, J. Adult stem cells at work: Regenerating skeletal muscle. *Cell Mol. Life Sci.* **2019**, *76*, 2559–2570.
360. Pajalunga, D.; Crescenzi, M. Restoring the Cell Cycle and Proliferation Competence in Terminally Differentiated Skeletal Muscle Myotubes. *Cells* **2021**, *10*, 2753.
361. Hart, M.L.; Izeta, A.; Herrera-Imbroda, B.; Amend, B.; Brinchmann, J.E. Cell Therapy for Stress Urinary Incontinence. *Tissue Eng. Part B Rev.* **2015**, *21*, 365–376.

362. Herrera-Imbroda, B.; Lara, M.F.; Izeta, A.; Sievert, K.D.; Hart, M.L. Stress urinary incontinence animal models as a tool to study cell-based regenerative therapies targeting the urethral sphincter. *Adv. Drug Deliv. Rev.* **2015**, *82–83*, 106–116.

363. Gotoh, M.; Yamamoto, T.; Shimizu, S.; Matsukawa, Y.; Kato, M.; Majima, T.; Takai, S.; Funahashi, Y.; Toriyama, K. Treatment of male stress urinary incontinence using autologous adipose-derived regenerative cells: Long-term efficacy and safety. *Int. J. Urol.* **2019**, *26*, 400–405.

364. Blaganje, M.; Lukanović, A. Intrasphincteric autologous myoblast injections with electrical stimulation for stress urinary incontinence. *Int. J. Gynaecol. Obstet.* **2012**, *117*, 164–167.

365. Aragón, I.M.; Imbroda, B.H.; Lara, M.F. Cell Therapy Clinical Trials for Stress Urinary Incontinence: Current Status and Perspectives. *Int. J. Med. Sci.* **2018**, *15*, 195–204.

366. Mitterberger, M.; Pinggera, G.M.; Marksteiner, R.; Margreiter, E.; Plattner, R.; Klima, G.; Strasser, H. Functional and histological changes after myoblast injections in the porcine rhabdosphincter. *Eur. Urol.* **2007**, *52*, 1736–1743.

367. Burdzinska, A.; Crayton, R.; Dybowski, B.; Idziak, M.; Gala, K.; Radziszewski, P.; Paczek, L. The effect of endoscopic administration of autologous porcine muscle-derived cells into the urethral sphincter. *Urology* **2013**, *82*, 743.e1–743.e8.

368. Burdzinska, A.; Dybowski, B.; Zarychta-Wisniewska, W.; Kulesza, A.; Zagozdzon, R.; Gajewski, Z.; Paczek, L. The Anatomy of Caprine Female Urethra and Characteristics of Muscle and Bone Marrow Derived Caprine Cells for Autologous Cell Therapy Testing. *Anat. Rec.* **2017**, *300*, 577–588.

369. Burdzinska, A.; Dybowski, B.; Zarychta-Wisniewska, W.; Kulesza, A.; Butrym, M.; Zagozdzon, R.; Graczyk-Jarzynka, A.; Radziszewski, P.; Gajewski, Z.; Paczek, L. Intraurethral co-transplantation of bone marrow mesenchymal stem cells and muscle-derived cells improves the urethral closure. *Stem Cell Res. Ther.* **2018**, *9*, 239.
370. Jankowski, R.J.; Deasy, B.M.; Huard, J. Muscle-derived stem cells. *Gene Ther.* **2002**, *9*, 642–647.
371. Mau, M.; Oksbjerg, N.; Rehfeldt, C. Establishment and conditions for growth and differentiation of a myoblast cell line derived from the semimembranosus muscle of newborn piglets. *In Vitro Cell. Dev. Biol.-Anim.* **2008**, *44*, 1–5.
372. Dezawa, M.; Ishikawa, H.; Itokazu, Y.; Yoshihara, T.; Hoshino, M.; Takeda, S.; Ide, C.; Nabeshima, Y. Bone marrow stromal cells generate muscle cells and repair muscle degeneration. *Science* **2005**, *309*, 314–317.
373. Yoshida, N.; Yoshida, S.; Koishi, K.; Masuda, K.; Nabeshima, Y. Cell heterogeneity upon myogenic differentiation: Down-regulation of MyoD and Myf-5 generates ‚reserve cells‘. *J. Cell Sci.* **1998**, *111 Pt 6*, 769–779.
374. Hannon, K.; Kudla, A.J.; McAvoy, M.J.; Clase, K.L.; Olwin, B.B. Differentially expressed fibroblast growth factors regulate skeletal muscle development through autocrine and paracrine mechanisms. *J. Cell Biol.* **1996**, *132*, 1151–1159.
375. Foster, A.A.; Marquardt, L.M.; Heilshorn, S.C. The Diverse Roles of Hydrogel Mechanics in Injectable Stem Cell Transplantation. *Curr. Opin. Chem. Eng.* **2017**, *15*, 15–23.
376. Sasca, D.; Szybinski, J.; Schuler, A.; Shah, V.; Heidelberger, J.; Haehnel, P.S.; Dolnik, A.; Kriege, O.; Fehr, E.M.; Gebhardt, W.H.; et al. NCAM1

(CD56) promotes leukemogenesis and confers drug resistance in AML. *Blood* **2019**, *133*, 2305–2319.

377. Gunasekara, C.J.; Scott, C.A.; Laritsky, E.; Baker, M.S.; MacKay, H.; Duryea, J.D.; Kessler, N.J.; Hellenthal, G.; Wood, A.C.; Hodges, K.R.; et al. A genomic atlas of systemic interindividual epigenetic variation in humans. *Genome Biol.* **2019**, *20*, 105.
378. Vinarov, A.; Atala, A.; Yoo, J.; Slusarenco, R.; Zhumataev, M.; Zhito, A.; Butnaru, D. Cell therapy for stress urinary incontinence: Present-day frontiers. *J. Tissue Eng. Regen. Med.* **2018**, *12*, e1108–e1121.
379. Whiting, D.; Hamdoon, M.; Sriprasad, S. Stem cell therapy for stress urinary incontinence. *J. Clin. Urol.* **2020**, *13*, 62–69.
380. Nriagu, J.O. A History of Global Metal Pollution. *Science* **1996**, *272*, 223–224.
381. Das, K.; Debacker, V.; Pillet, S.; Bouquegneau, J.M. Heavy Metals in Marine Mammals. In *Toxicology of Marine Mammals*, 1st ed.; Vos, J.V., Bossart, G.D., Fournier, M., O'Shea, T., Eds.; Taylor and Francis Publishers: Washington, DC, USA, 2003; Volume 1, pp. 135–167.
382. Roy, S.P. Overview of heavy metals and aquatic environment with notes on their recovery. *Ecoscan* **2010**, *4*, 235–240.
383. Apostoli, P. Elements in Environmental and Occupational Medicine. *J. Chromatogr. B* **2002**, *778*, 63–97.
384. Kunito, T.; Nakamura, S.; Ikemoto, T.; Anan, Y.; Kubota, R.; Tanabe, S.; Rosas, F.C.W.; Fillmann, G.; Readman, J.W. Concentration and Subcellular Distribution of Trace Elements in Liver of Small Cetaceans Incidentally Caught along the Brazilian Coast. *Mar. Pollut. Bull.* **2004**, *49*, 574–587.

385. Stavros, H.C.; Stolen, M.; Durden, W.N.; McFee, W.; Bossart, G.D.; Fair, P.A. Correlation and Toxicological Inference of Trace Elements in Tissues from Stranded and Free-Ranging Bottlenose Dolphins (*Tursiops truncatus*). *Chemosphere* **2011**, *82*, 1649–1661.
386. Bossart, G.D. Marine Mammals as Sentinel Species for Oceans and Human Health. *Vet. Pathol.* **2011**, *48*, 676–690.
387. Agusa, T.; Nomura, K.; Kunito, T.; Anan, Y.; Iwata, H.; Miyazaki, N.; Tatsukawa, R.; Tanabe, S. Interelement Relationships and Age-Related Variation of Trace Element Concentrations in Liver of Striped Dolphins (*Stenella coeruleoalba*) from Japanese Coastal Waters. *Mar. Pollut. Bull.* **2008**, *57*, 807–815.
388. Yasuda, Y.; Horai, S.; Itai, T.; Isobe, T.; Matsuishi, T.; Yamada, T.; Tajima, Y.; Takahashi, S.; Tanabe, S. A Comparative Study on Temporal Trends of Trace Elements in Harbor Porpoise (*Phocoena phocoena*) from Coastal Waters of North Japan. *Interdiscip. Stud. Environ. Chem.* **2012**, *6*, 151–159.
389. Law, R.J.; Morris, R.J.; Allchin, C.R.; Jones, B.R.; Nicholson, M.D. Metals and Organochlorines in Small Cetaceans Stranded on the East Coast of Australia. *Mar. Pollut. Bull.* **2003**, *46*, 1206–1211.
390. Butterfield, N.; Gaylard, S. *The Heavy Metal Status of South Australian Dolphins: An Overview*; Environment Protection Authority: Adelaide, Australia, 2005.
391. Lavery, T.J.; Butterfield, N.; Kemper, C.M.; Reid, R.J.; Sanderson, K. Metals and Selenium in the Liver and Bone of Three Dolphin Species from South Australia, 1988–2004. *Sci. Total Environ.* **2008**, *390*, 77–85
392. Lavery, T.J.; Kemper, C.M.; Sanderson, K.; Schultz, C.G.; Coyle, P.; Mitchell, J.G.; Seuront, L. Heavy Metal Toxicity of Kidney and Bone Tissues

in South Australian Adult Bottlenose Dolphins (*Tursiops aduncus*). *Mar. Environ. Res.* **2009**, *67*, 1–7.

393. Stockin, K.A.; Law, R.J.; Duignan, P.J.; Jones, G.W.; Porter, L.; Mirimin, L.; Meynier, L.; Orams, M.B. Trace Elements, PCBs and Organochlorine Pesticides in New Zealand Common Dolphins (*Delphinus* sp.). *Sci. Total Environ.* **2007**, *387*, 333–345.
394. Stavros, H.C.; Bossart, G.D.; Hulsey, T.C.; Fair, P.A. Trace element concentrations in blood of free-ranging bottlenose dolphins (*Tursiops truncatus*): Influence of age, sex and location. *Mar. Pollut. Bull.* **2008**, *56*, 371–379.
395. Cáceres-Saez, I.; Ribeiro Guevara, S.; Dellabianca, N.A.; Goodall, R.N.; Cappozzo, H.L. Heavy Metals and Essential Elements in Commerson‘s Dolphins (*Cephalorhynchus c. commersonii*) from the Southwestern South Atlantic Ocean. *Environ. Monit. Assess.* **2013**, *185*, 5375–5386.
396. Frodello, J.P.; Viale, D.; Marchand, B. Metal Concentrations in the Milk and Tissues of a Nursing *Tursiops truncatus* Female. *Mar. Pollut. Bull.* **2002**, *44*, 551–554.
397. Lahaye, V.; Bustamante, P.; Law, R.J.; Learmonth, J.A.; Santos, M.B.; Boon, J.P.; Rogan, E.; Dabin, W.; Addink, M.; López, A.; et al. Biological and Ecological Factors Related to Trace Element Levels in Harbour Porpoises (*Phocoena phocoena*) from European Waters. *Mar. Environ. Res.* **2007**, *64*, 247–266.
398. Cardellicchio, N.; Giandomenico, S.; Ragone, P.; Di Leo, A. Tissue Distribution of Metals in Striped Dolphins (*Stenella coeruleoalba*) from the Apulian Coasts, Southern Italy. *Mar. Environ. Res.* **2000**, *49*, 55–66.

399. Capelli, R.; Das, K.; Pellegrini, R.D.; Drava, G.; Lepoint, G.; Miglio, C.; Minganti, V.; Poggi, R. Distribution of Trace Elements in Organs of Six Species of Cetaceans from the Ligurian Sea (Mediterranean), and the Relationship with Stable Carbon and Nitrogen Ratios. *Sci. Total Environ.* **2008**, *390*, 569–578.
400. Shoham-Frider, E.; Amiel, S.; Roditi-Elasar, M.; Kress, N. Risso's Dolphin (*Grampus griseus*) Stranding on the Coast of Israel (Eastern Mediterranean). Autopsy Results and Trace Metal Concentrations. *Sci. Total Environ.* **2002**, *295*, 157–166.
401. Roditi-Elasar, M.; Kerem, D.; Hornung, H.; Kress, N.; Shoham-Frider, E.; Goffman, O.; Spanier, E. Heavy metal levels in bottlenose and striped dolphins off the Mediterranean coast of Israel. *Mar. Pollut. Bull.* **2003**, *46*, 503–512.
402. Das, K.; Siebert, U.; Fontaine, M.; Jauniaux, T.; Holsbeek, L.; Bouquegneau, J.M. Ecological and Pathological Factors Related to Trace Metal Concentrations in Harbour Porpoises (*Phocoena phocoena*) from the North Sea and Adjacent Areas. *Mar. Ecol. Prog. Ser.* **2004**, *281*, 283–295.
403. Galov, A.; Lauc, G.; Nikolić, N.; Šatović, Z.; Gomerčić, T.; Đuras Gomerčić, M.; Kocijan, I.; Šeol, B.; Gomerčić, H. Records and Genetic Diversity of Striped Dolphins (*Stenella coeruleoalba*) from the Croatian Coast of the Adriatic Sea. *Mar. Biodivers. Rec.* **2009**, *2*, e98.
404. Pompe-Gotal, J.; Srebočan, E.; Gomerčić, H.; Prevendar Crnić, A. Mercury Concentrations in the Tissues of Bottlenose Dolphins (*Tursiops truncatus*) and Striped Dolphins (*Stenella coeruleoalba*) Stranded on the Croatian Adriatic Coast. *Vet. Med. Czech* **2009**, *54*, 598–604.

405. Bilandžić, N.; Sedak, M.; Đokić, M.; Đuras Gomerčić, M.; Gomerčić, T.; Zadravec, M.; Benić, M.; Prevendar Crnić, A. Toxic Element Concentrations in the Bottlenose (*Tursiops truncatus*), Striped (*Stenella coeruleoalba*), and Risso's (*Grampus griseus*) Dolphins Stranded in Eastern Adriatic Sea. *Bull. Environ. Contam. Toxicol.* **2012**, *89*, 467–473.
406. Šuran, J.; Đuras, M.; Gomerčić, T.; Bilandžić, N.; Prevendar Crnić, A. Cadmium and Lead Concentrations in the Tissues of Bottlenose Dolphins (*Tursiops truncatus*) and Striped Dolphins (*Stenella coeruleoalba*) Stranded on the Croatian Adriatic Coast. *Vet. Arhiv* **2015**, *85*, 677–688
407. Bilandžić, N.; Sedak, M.; Đokić, M.; Đuras, M.; Gomerčić, T.; Benić, M.; Šimić, B. Concentration of Mercury and Selenium in Tissues of Five Cetacean Species from Croatian Coastal Waters. *Arch. Biol. Sci.* **2015**, *67*, 1377–1389.
408. Sedak, M.; Bilandžić, N.; Đokić, M.; Đuras, M.; Gomerčić, T.; Benić, M. Body Burdens and Distribution of Mercury and Selenium in Bottlenose, Striped and Risso's Dolphins along the Adriatic Coast: A 20-Year Retrospective. *Mar. Pollut. Bull.* **2022**, *185*, 114298.
409. Sedak, M.; Đokić, M.; Bilandžić, N.; Gomerčić, T.; Benić, M.; Zadravec, M.; Đuras, M. Cetacean Species Found Stranded along Croatian Coast of the Adriatic Sea as Bioindicators of Non-Essential Trace Elements in the Environment. *Aquat. Toxicol.* **2025**, *279*, 107206.
410. Bilandžić, N.; Đokić, M.; Sedak, M.; Đuras, M.; Gomerčić, T.; Benić, M. Copper Levels in Tissues of Dolphins Tursiops truncatus, Stenella coeruleoalba and Grampus griseus from the Croatian Adriatic Sea. *Bull. Environ. Contam. Toxicol.* **2016**, *97*, 367–373.

411. Đokić, M.; Bilandžić, N.; Sedak, M.; Đuras, M.; Gomerčić, T.; Benić, M.; Bolanča, T. Manganese Concentrations in Tissues and Skin of Three Dolphin Species Stranded in the Croatian Waters of the Adriatic Sea from 1995 to 2013. *Bull. Environ. Contam. Toxicol.* **2018**, *100*, 317–323.
412. Beck, K.M.; Fair, P.; McFee, W.; Wolf, D. Heavy Metals in Livers of Bottlenose Dolphins Stranded along the South Carolina Coast. *Mar. Pollut. Bull.* **1997**, *34*, 734–739.
413. Slooten, E. Age, Growth, and Reproduction in Hector's Dolphins. *Can. J. Zool.* **1991**, *69*, 1689–1700.
414. Hohn, A.A.; Scott, M.D.; Wells, R.S.; Sweeney, J.C.; Irvine, A.B. Growth Layers in Teeth from Known-Age, Free-Ranging Bottlenose Dolphins. *Mar. Mammal Sci.* **1989**, *5*, 315–342.
415. Andre, J.; Boudou, A.; Ribeyre, F.; Bernhard, M. Comparative Study of Mercury Accumulation in Dolphins (*Stenella coeruleoalba*) from French Atlantic and Mediterranean Coasts. *Sci. Total Environ.* **1991**, *104*, 191–209.
416. Becker, P.R.; Mackey, E.A.; Demiralp, R.; Suydam, R.; Early, G.; Koster, B.J.; Wise, S.A. Relationship of Silver with Selenium and Mercury in the Liver of Two Species of Toothed Whales (Odontocetes). *Mar. Pollut. Bull.* **1995**, *30*, 262–271.
417. Wagemann, R.; Muir, D. Concentrations of Heavy Metals and Organochlorines in Marine Mammals of Northern Waters: Overview and Evaluation. *Can. Tech. Rep. Fish. Aquat. Sci.* **1984**, 1–97.
418. Eisler, R. Copper. In *Handbook of Chemical Risk Assessment*, 1st ed.; Eisler, R., Ed.; Lewis Publishers: Boca Raton, FL, USA, 2000; Volume 1, pp. 127–235.

419. O'Shea, T.J.; Moore, J.F.; Kochman, H.I. Contaminant Concentrations in Manatees in Florida. *J. Wildl. Manag.* **1984**, *48*, 741–748
420. Bellante, A.; Sprovieri, M.; Buscaino, G.; Manta, D.S.; Buffa, G.; Di Stefano, V.; Bonanno, A.; Barra, M.; Patti, B.; Giacoma, C.; et al. Trace Elements and Vanadium in Tissues and Organs of Five Species of Cetaceans from Italian Coasts. *Chem. Ecol.* **2009**, *25*, 311–323.
421. Frodello, J.P.; Marchand, B. Cadmium, Copper, Lead, and Zinc in Five Toothed Whale Species of the Mediterranean Sea. *Int. J. Toxicol.* **2001**, *20*, 339–343.
422. Holsbeek, L.; Siebert, U.; Joiris, C.R. Heavy Metals in Dolphins Stranded on the French Atlantic Coast. *Sci. Total Environ.* **1998**, *217*, 241–249.
423. Shoham-Frider, E.; Kress, N.; Wynne, D.; Scheinin, A.; Roditi-Elsar, M.; Kerem, D. Persistent Organochlorine Pollutants and Heavy Metals in Tissues of Common Bottlenose Dolphin (*Tursiops truncatus*) from the Levantine Basin of the Eastern Mediterranean. *Chemosphere* **2009**, *77*, 621–627.
424. Capelli, R.; Drava, G.; De Pellegrini, R.; Minganti, V.; Poggi, R. Study of Trace Elements in Organs and Tissues of Striped Dolphins (*Stenella coeruleoalba*) Found Dead along the Ligurian Coasts (Italy). *Adv. Environ. Res.* **2000**, *4*, 31–34.
425. Monaci, F.; Borrel, A.; Leonzio, C.; Marsili, L.; Calzada, N. Trace Elements in Striped Dolphins (*Stenella coeruleoalba*) from the Western Mediterranean. *Environ. Pollut.* **1998**, *99*, 61–68.
426. Cardellicchio, N.; Decataldo, A.; Di Leo, A.; Giandomenico, S. Trace Elements in Organs and Tissues of Striped Dolphins (*Stenella coeruleoalba*) from the Mediterranean Sea (Southern Italy). *Chemosphere* **2002**, *49*, 85–90.

427. Wafo, E.; Risoul, V.; Schembri, T.; Lagadec, V.; Dhermain, F.; Mama, C.; Boissery, P.; Portugal, H. Methylmercury and Trace Element Distribution in the Organs of *Stenella coeruleoalba* Dolphins Stranded on the French Mediterranean Coast. *Open Environ. Sci.* **2014**, *8*, 35–48.
428. Borrell, A.; Clusa, M.; Aguilar, A.; Drago, M. Use of Epidermis for the Monitoring of Tissular Trace Elements in Mediterranean Striped Dolphins (*Stenella coeruleoalba*). *Chemosphere* **2015**, *122*, 288–294.
429. Rojo-Nieto, E.; Fernández-Maldonado, C. Assessing trace elements in striped dolphins from the Strait of Gibraltar: Clues to link the bioaccumulation in the westernmost Mediterranean Sea area and nearest Atlantic Ocean. *Chemosphere* **2017**, *170*, 41–50.
430. Shoham-Frider, E.; Goffman, O.; Harlavan, Y.; Kress, N.; Morick, D.; Roditi-Elasar, M.; Shefer, E.; Kerem, D. Trace Elements in Striped Dolphins (*Stenella coeruleoalba*) from the Eastern Mediterranean: A 10-Years Perspective. *Mar. Pollut. Bull.* **2016**, *109*, 624–632.
431. Shoham-Frider, E.; Kerem, D.; Roditi-Elasar, M.; Goffman, O.; Morick, D.; Yoffe, O.; Kress, N. Trace Elements in Tissues of Cetacean Species Rarely Stranded along the Israeli Mediterranean Coast. *Mar. Pollut. Bull.* **2014**, *83*, 376–382.
432. Law, R.J.; Fileman, C.F.; Hopkins, A.D.; Baker, J.R.; Harwood, J.; Jackson, D.B.; Kennedy, S.; Martin, A.R.; Morris, R.J. Concentrations of Trace Metals in the Livers of Marine Mammals (Seals, Porpoises and Dolphins) from Waters Around the British Isles. *Mar. Pollut. Bull.* **1991**, *22*, 183–191.
433. Carvalho, M.L.; Pereira, R.A.; Brito, J. Heavy Metals in Soft Tissues of *Tursiops truncatus* and *Delphinus delphis* from the West Atlantic Ocean by X-Ray Spectrometry. *Sci. Total Environ.* **2002**, *292*, 247–254.

434. Aubail, A.; Méndez-Fernandez, P.; Bustamante, P.; Churlaud, C.; Ferreira, M.; Vingada, J.V.; Caurant, F. Use of Skin and Blubber Tissues of Small Cetaceans to Assess the Trace Element Content of Internal Organs. *Mar. Pollut. Bull.* **2013**, *76*, 158–169.
435. Morris, R.J.; Law, R.J.; Allchin, C.R.; Kelly, C.A.; Fileman, C.F. Metals and Organochlorines in Dolphins and Porpoises of Cardigan Bay, West Wales. *Mar. Pollut. Bull.* **1989**, *20*, 512–523.
436. Meador, J.P.; Ernest, D.; Hohn, A.A.; Tilbury, K.; Gorzelany, J.; Worthy, G.; Stein, J.E. Comparison of Elements in Bottlenose Dolphins Stranded on the Beaches of Texas and Florida in the Gulf of Mexico over a One-Year Period. *Arch. Environ. Contam. Toxicol.* **1999**, *36*, 87–98.
437. Stavros, H.C.; Bossart, G.D.; Hulsey, T.C.; Fair, P.A. Trace Element Concentrations in Skin of Free-Ranging Bottlenose Dolphins (*Tursiops truncatus*) from the Southeast Atlantic Coast. *Sci. Total Environ.* **2007**, *388*, 300–315.
438. Lemos, L.S.; de Moura, J.F.; Hauser-Davis, R.A.; de Campos, R.C.; Siciliano, S. Small Cetaceans Found Stranded or Accidentally Captured in Southeastern Brazil: Bioindicators of Essential and Non-Essential Trace Elements in the Environment. *Ecotoxicol. Environ. Saf.* **2013**, *97*, 166–175.
439. Hansen, A.M.; Bryan, C.E.; West, K.L.; Jensen, B.A. Trace Element Concentrations in Liver of 16 Species of Cetaceans Stranded on Pacific Islands from 1997 through 2013. *Arch. Environ. Contam. Toxicol.* **2015**, *70*, 75–95.
440. Monteiro, S.S.; Torres, J.; Ferreira, M.; Marçalo, A.; Nicolau, L.; Vingada, J.V.; Eira, C. Ecological Variables Influencing Trace Element Concentrations

in Bottlenose Dolphins (*Tursiops truncatus*, Montagu 1821) Stranded in Continental Portugal. *Sci. Total Environ.* **2016**, *544*, 837–844.

441. Honda, K.; Tatsukawa, R. Distribution of Cadmium and Zinc in Tissues and Organs, and Their Age-Related Changes in Striped Dolphins, *Stenella coeruleoalba*. *Arch. Environ. Contam. Toxicol.* **1983**, *12*, 543–550.

442. Storelli, M.M.; Marcotrigiano, G.O. Environmental Contamination in Bottlenose Dolphin (*Tursiops truncatus*): Relationship between Levels of Metals, Methylmercury, and Organochlorine Compounds in an Adult Female, Her Neonate, and a Calf. *Bull. Environ. Contam. Toxicol.* **2000**, *64*, 333–340.

443. Fujise, Y.; Honda, K.; Tatsukawa, R.; Mishima, S. Tissue Distribution of Heavy Metals in Dall's Porpoise in the Northwestern Pacific. *Mar. Pollut. Bull.* **1988**, *19*, 226–230.

444. Law, R.J.; Jones, B.R.; Baker, J.R.; Kennedy, S.; Milne, R.L.; Morris, R.J. Trace Metals in the Livers of Marine Mammals from the Welsh Coast and the Irish Sea. *Mar. Pollut. Bull.* **1992**, *24*, 296–304.

445. Law, R.J. Metals in Marine Mammals. In *Environmental Contaminants in Wildlife: Interpreting Tissue Concentrations*, 1st ed.; Beyer, W., Heinz, G., Redmon-Norwood, A., Eds.; CRC Lewis Publishers: Boca Raton, FL, USA, 1996; pp. 357–376.

446. Yang, J.; Kunito, T.; Anan, Y.; Tanabe, S.; Miyazaki, N. Total and Subcellular Distribution of Trace Elements in the Liver of a Mother–Fetus Pair of Dall's Porpoises (*Phocoenoides dalli*). *Mar. Pollut. Bull.* **2004**, *48*, 1122–1129.

447. Lahaye, V.; Bustamante, P.; Dabin, W.; Churlaud, C.; Caurant, F. Trace Element Levels in Foetus-Mother Pairs of Short-Beaked Common Dolphins

(*Delphinus delphis*) Stranded Along the French Coasts. *Environ. Int.* **2007**, *33*, 1021–1028.

448. Teigen, S.; Andersen, R.; Daae, H.; Skaare, J. Heavy Metal Content in Liver and Kidneys of Grey Seals (*Halichoerus grypus*) in Various Life Stages Correlated with Metallothionein Levels: Some Metal—Binding Characteristics of This Protein. *Environ. Toxicol. Chem.* **2009**, *18*, 2364–2369.
449. Robbins, D.T. *Wildlife Feeding and Nutrition*; Academic: San Diego, CA, USA, 1983.
450. Mackey, E.A.; Oflaz, R.; Epstein, M.S.; Buehler, B.; Porter, B.J.; Rowles, T.K.; Wise, S.A.; Becker, P.R. Elemental Composition of Liver and Kidney Tissues of Rough-Toothed Dolphins (*Steno bredanensis*). *Arch. Environ. Contam. Toxicol.* **2003**, *44*, 523–532.
451. Bellante, A.; Manta, D.S.; Traina, A.; Buscaino, G.; Buffa, G.; Barra, M.; Tamburrino, S.; Mazzola, S.; Sprovieri, M. Trace Elements in Tissues of Sperm Whales Stranded along the Italian Coast. *Chem. Ecol.* **2013**, *29*, 404–414.
452. Julshamn, K.; Andersen, A.; Ringdal, O.; Mørkøre, J. Trace Elements Intake in the Faroe Islands. I. Element Levels in Edible Parts of Pilot Whales (*Globicephalus meleanus*). *Sci. Total Environ.* **1987**, *65*, 53–62.
453. Poldan, I. *Analysis of the Jaw (Cephalopoda) from the Stomachs of Bottlenose Dolphins (Tursiops truncatus) from the Adriatic Sea*; Student Work; Faculty of Veterinary Medicine; University of Zagreb: Zagreb, Croatia, 2004.
454. Honda, K.; Tatsukawa, R.; Itano, K.; Miyazaki, N.; Fujiyama, T. Heavy Metal Concentrations in Muscle, Liver, and Kidney Tissue of Striped

Dolphin, *Stenella coeruleoalba*, and Their Variations with Body Length, Weight, Age, and Sex. *Agric. Biol. Chem.* **1983**, *47*, 1219–1228.

455. Emonet-Piccardi, N.; Richard, M.J.; Ravanat, J.L.; Signorini, N.; Cadet, J.; Béani, J.C. Protective Effects of Antioxidants against UVA-Induced DNA Damage in Human Skin Fibroblasts in Culture. *Free Radic. Res.* **1998**, *29*, 307–313.
456. Bennett, P.M.; Jepson, P.D.; Law, R.J.; Jones, B.R.; Kuiken, T.; Baker, J.R.; Rogan, E.; Kirkwood, J.K. Exposure to Heavy Metals and Infectious Disease Mortality in Harbour Porpoises from England and Wales. *Environ. Pollut.* **2001**, *112*, 33–40.
457. Noda, K.; Ichihashi, H.; Loughlin, T.R.; Baba, N.; Kiyota, M.; Tatsukawa, R. Distribution of Heavy Metals in Muscle, Liver and Kidney of Northern Fur Seal (*Callorhinus ursinus*) Caught off Sanriku, Japan and from the Pribilof Islands, Alaska. *Environ. Pollut.* **1995**, *90*, 51–59.
458. Watanabe, I.; Ichihashi, H.; Tanabe, S.; Amano, M.; Miyazaki, N.; Petrov, E.A.; Tatsukawa, R. Trace Element Accumulation in Baikal Seal (*Phoca sibirica*) from Lake Baikal. *Environ. Pollut.* **1996**, *94*, 169–179.
459. Anan, Y.; Kunito, T.; Ikemoto, T.; Kubota, R.; Watanabe, I.; Tanabe, S.; Miyazaki, N.; Petrov, E.A. Elevated Concentrations of Trace Elements in Caspian Seals (*Phoca caspica*) Found Stranded during the Mass Mortality Events in 2000. *Arch. Environ. Contam. Toxicol.* **2002**, *42*, 354–362.
460. Davis, G.K. Microelement Interactions of Zinc, Copper, and Iron in Mammalian Species. *Ann. N. Y. Acad. Sci.* **1980**, *355*, 130–139
461. Zhou, J.L.; Salvador, S.M.; Liu, Y.P.; Sequeira, M. Heavy Metals in the Tissues of Common Dolphins (*Delphinus delphis*) Stranded on the Portuguese Coast. *Sci. Total Environ.* **2001**, *273*, 61–76.

462. Pacyna, J.M.; Pacyna, E.G. An Assessment of Global and Regional Emissions of Trace Metals to the Atmosphere from Anthropogenic Sources Worldwide. *Environ. Rev.* **2001**, *9*, 269–298.

463. Bargagli, R. Trace Metals in Antarctic Organisms and the Development of Circumpolar Biomonitoring Networks. *Rev. Environ. Contam. Toxicol.* **2001**, *171*, 53–110.

464. Kubota, R.; Kunito, T.; Tanabe, S. Arsenic Accumulation in the Liver Tissue of Marine Mammals. *Environ. Pollut.* **2001**, *115*, 303–312.

465. Watanabe, I.; Kunito, T.; Tanabe, S.; Amano, M.; Koyama, Y.; Miyazaki, N.; Petrov, E.A.; Tatsukawa, R. Accumulation of Heavy Metals in Caspian Seals (*Phoca caspica*). *Arch. Environ. Contam. Toxicol.* **2002**, *43*, 109–120.

466. Yoshitome, R.; Kunito, T.; Ikemoto, T.; Tanabe, S.; Zenke, H.; Yamauchi, M.; Miyazaki, N. Global Distribution of Radionuclides (^137Cs and ^40K) in Marine Mammals. *Environ. Sci. Technol.* **2003**, *37*, 4597–4602.

467. Agusa, T.; Nomura, K.; Kunito, T.; Anan, Y.; Iwata, H.; Tanabe, S. Accumulation of Trace Elements in Harp Seals (Phoca groenlandica) from Pangnirtung in the Baffin Island, Canada. *Mar. Pollut. Bull.* **2011**, *63*, 489–499.

468. Muir, D.C.; Wagemann, R.; Grift, N.P.; Norstrom, R.J.; Simon, M.; Lien, J. Organochlorine Chemical and Heavy Metal Contaminants in White-Beaked Dolphins (*Lagenorhynchus albirostris*) and Pilot Whales (*Globicephala melaena*) from the Coast of Newfoundland, Canada. *Arch. Environ. Contam. Toxicol.* **1988**, *17*, 613–629.

469. Koury, J.C.; Donangelo, C.M. Zinco, Estresse Oxidativo e Atividade Física. *Rev. Nutr.* **2003**, *16*, 433–441.

470. Kunito, T.; Watanabe, I.; Yasunaga, G.; Fujise, Y.; Tanabe, S. Using Trace Elements in Skin to Discriminate the Populations of Minke Whales in Southern Hemisphere. *Mar. Environ. Res.* **2002**, *53*, 175–197.
471. Ciesielski, T.M.; Pastukhov, M.V.; Fodor, P.; Bertenyi, Z.; Namieśnik, J.; Szefer, P. Relationships and Bioaccumulation of Chemical Elements in the Baikal Seal (*Phoca sibirica*). *Environ. Pollut.* **2006**, *139*, 372–384.
472. Griesel, S.; Mundry, R.; Kakuschke, A.; Fonfara, S.; Siebert, U.; Prange, A. Mineral Elements and Essential Trace Elements in Blood of Seals of the North Sea Measured by Total-Reflection X-Ray Fluorescence Analysis. *Spectrochim. Acta Part B* **2006**, *61*, 1158–1165.
473. Stockham, S.; Scott, M.A. Proteins. In *Fundamentals of Veterinary Clinical Pathology*, 2nd ed.; Stockham, S., Scott, M.A., Eds.; Blackwell Publishing: Oxford, UK, 2008; pp. 370–405.
474. Bossuyt, P.M.; Reitsma, J.B.; Bruns, D.E.; Gatsonis, C.A.; Glasziou, P.P.; Irwig, L.M.; Lijmer, J.G.; Moher, D.; Rennie, D.; de Vet, H.C.W. Towards complete and accurate reporting of studies of diagnostic accuracy: The STARD initiative. *Vet. Clin. Pathol.* **2007**, *36*, 8–12.
475. Roudiere, L.; Boularan, A.M.; Bonardet, A.; Vallat, C.; Cristol, J.P.; Dupuy, A.M. Evaluation of a capillary zone electrophoresis system versus a conventional agarose gel system for routine serum protein separation and monoclonal component typing. *Clin. Lab.* **2006**, *52*, 19–27.
476. Abate, O.; Zanatta, R.; Malisano, T.; Dotta, U. Canine serum protein patterns using high-resolution electrophoresis (HRE). *Vet. J.* **2000**, *159*, 154–160.

477. Robeck, T.R.; Nollens, H.H. Hematological and serum biochemical analytes reflect physiological challenges during gestation and lactation in killer whales (*Orcinus orca*). *Zoo Biol.* **2013**, *32*, 497–509.

478. Tryland, M.; Brun, E. Serum chemistry of the minke whale from the northeastern Atlantic. *J. Wildl. Dis.* **2001**, *37*, 332–341.

479. St. Aubin, D.J.; Forney, K.A.; Chivers, S.J.; Scott, M.D.; Danil, K.; Romano, T.A.; Wells, R.S.; Gulland, F.M.D. Hematological, serum, and plasma chemical constituents in pantropical spotted dolphins (*Stenella attenuata*) following chase, encirclement, and tagging. *Mar. Mammal Sci.* **2013**, *29*, 14–35.

480. Tryland, M.; Thoresen, S.I.; Kovacs, K.M.; Lydersen, C. Serum chemistry of free-ranging white whales (*Delphinapterus leucas*) in Svalbard. *Vet. Clin. Pathol.* **2006**, *35*, 199–203.

481. Greig, D.J.; Gulland, F.M.D.; Rios, C.A.; Hall, A.J. Hematology and serum chemistry in stranded and wild-caught harbor seals in central California: Reference intervals, predictors of survival, and parameters affecting blood variables. *J. Wildl. Dis.* **2010**, *46*, 1172–1184.

482. Tryland, M.; Lydersen, C.; Kovacs, K.M.; Thoresen, S.I. Serum chemistry reference values in free-ranging north Atlantic male walruses *(Odobenus rosmarus rosmarus)* from the Svalbard archipelago. *Vet. Clin. Pathol.* **2009**, *38*, 501–506.

483. Geffré, A.; Friedrichs, K.; Harr, K.; Concordet, D.; Trumel, C.; Braun, J.P. Reference values: A review. *Vet. Clin. Pathol.* **2009**, *38*, 288–298.

484. Schwacke, L.H.; Hall, A.J.; Townsend, F.I.; Wells, R.S.; Hansen, L.J.; Hohn, A.A.; Bossart, G.D.; Fair, P.A.; Rowles, T.K. Hematologic and serum biochemical reference intervals for free-ranging common bottlenose

dolphins (*Tursiops truncatus*) and variation in the istributions of clinicopathological valus related to geographic sampling site. *Am. J. Vet. Res.* **2009**, *70*, 973–985.

485. Gili, C.; Bonsembiante, F.; Bonanni, R.; Giordano, A.; Ledda, S.; Beffagna, G.; Paltrinieri, S.; Sommer, M.; Gelain, M.E. Detection of hereditary bisalbuminemia in bottlenose dolphins (*Tursiops truncatus*, Montagu 1821): Comparison between capillary zone and agarose gel electrophoresis. *BMC Vet. Res.* **2016**, *12*, 172.
486. Flower, J.E.; Langan, J.N.; Wells, R.S.; Cray, C.; Arheart, K.; Chinnadurai, S.K.; Adkesson, M.J. Serum acute-phase proteins in bottlenose dolphins (*Tursiops truncatus*) and correlation with commonly utilized inflammatory indices. *J. Zoo Wildl. Med.* **2020**, *51*, 657–662.
487. Giordano, A.; Paltrinieri, S. Interpretation of capillary zone electrophoresis compared with cellulose acetate and agarose gel electrophoresis: Reference intervals and diagnostic efficiency in dogs and cats. *Vet. Clin. Pathol.* **2010**, *39*, 464–473.
488. Geffré, A.; Concordet, D.; Braun, J.P.; Trumel, C. Reference Value Advisor: A new freeware set of macroinstructions to calculate reference intervals with Microsoft Excel. *Vet. Clin. Pathol.* **2011**, *40*, 107–112.
489. Friedrichs, K.R.; Harr, K.E.; Freeman, K.P.; Szladovits, B.; Walton, R.M.; Barnhart, K.F.; Blanco-Chavez, J. ASVCP reference interval guidelines: Determination of de novo reference intervals in veterinary species and other related topics. *Vet. Clin. Pathol.* **2012**, *41*, 441–453.
490. Cray, C. Protein electrophoresis of non-traditional species: A review. *Vet. Clin. Pathol.* **2021**, *50*, 478–494.

491. Levin, M. Marine Mammal Immunology. In *CRC Handbook of Marine Mammal Medicine*, 3rd ed.; Galland, F.M.D., Dierauf, L.A., Whitman, K.L., Eds.; CRC Press: Boca Raton, FL, USA, 2018; pp. 209–229.
492. Johnson, H.L.; Chiou, C.C.; Cho, C.T. Applications of acute phase reactants in infectious diseases. *J. Microbiol. Immunol. Infect.* **1999**, *32*, 73–82.
493. Cray, C.; Zaias, J.; Altman, N.H. Acute phase response in animals: A review. *Comp. Med.* **2009**, *59*, 517–526.
494. Profeta, F.; Di Francesco, C.E.; Marsilio, F.; Mignone, W.; Di Nocera, F.; De Carlo, E.; Lucifora, G.; Pietroluongo, G.; Baffoni, M.; Cocumelli, C.; et al. Retrospective seroepidemiological investigations against *Morbillivirus*, *Toxoplasma gondii* and *Brucella* spp. in Cetaceans stranded along the Italian coastline (1998–2014). *Res. Vet. Sci.* **2015**, *101*, 89–92.
495. Gelain, M.E.; Bonsembiante, F. Acute phase proteins in marine mammals: State of art, perspectives and challenges. *Front. Immunol.* **2019**, *10*, 1220.
496. Bossuyt, X.; Lissoir, B.; Mariën, G.; Maisin, D.; Vunckx, J.; Blanckaert, N.; Wallemacq, P. Automated serum protein electrophoresis by Capillarys. *Clin. Chem. Lab. Med.* **2003**, *41*, 704–710.
497. Jabeen, R.; Payne, D.; Wiktorowicz, J.; Mohammad, A.; Petersen, J. Capillary electrophoresis and the clinical laboratory. *Electrophoresis* **2006**, *27*, 2413–2438.
498. Gili, C.; Bonsembiante, F.; Beffagna, G.; Mazzariol, S.; Gelain, M.E. Mutations and polymorphism in albumin gene of bottlenose dolphin (*Tursiops truncatus*, Montagu 1821): First identification of mutations responsible of inherited bisalbuminemia. *Res. Vet. Sci.* **2017**, *114*, 12–17.

499. Zaias, J.; Bossart, G.D.; Cray, C. Comparison of agarose gel electrophoresis and capillary zone electrophoresis methods using serum from bottlenose dolphins (*Tursiops truncatus*). *Aquat. Mamm.* **2021**, *47*, 146–152.
500. Crivellente, F.; Bonato, M.; Cristofori, P. Analysis of mouse, rat, dog, marmoset, and human serum proteins by capillary electrophoresis: Comparison with agarose gel electrophoresis. *Vet. Clin. Pathol.* **2008**, *37*, 73–78.
501. Allender, M.C.; Junge, R.E.; Baker-Wylie, S.; Hileman, E.T.; Faust, L.J.; Cray, C. Plasma electrophoretic profiles in the eastern Massasauga (*Sistrurus catenatus*) and influences of age, sex, year, location, and snake fungal disease. *J. Zoo Wildl. Med.* **2015**, *46*, 767–773.
502. Flower, J.E.; Byrd, J.; Cray, C.; Allender, M.C. Plasma electrophoretic profiles and hemoglobin binding protein reference intervals in the eastern box turtle (*Terrapene carolina carolina*) and influences of age, sex, season, and location. *J. Zoo Wildl. Med.* **2014**, *45*, 836–842.
503. Wernick, M.B.; Martin-Jurado, O.; Beaufrère, H.; Howard, J.; Samour, J. Serum protein electrophoresis reference values in the gyrfalcon (*Falco rusticolus*). *Comp. Clin. Path.* **2018**, *27*, 493–497.
504. Freeman, K.P.; Baral, R.M.; Dhand, N.K.; Nielsen, S.S.; Jensen, A.L. Recommendations for designing and conducting veterinary clinical pathology biologic variation studies. *Vet. Clin. Pathol.* **2017**, *46*, 211–220.

About Authors

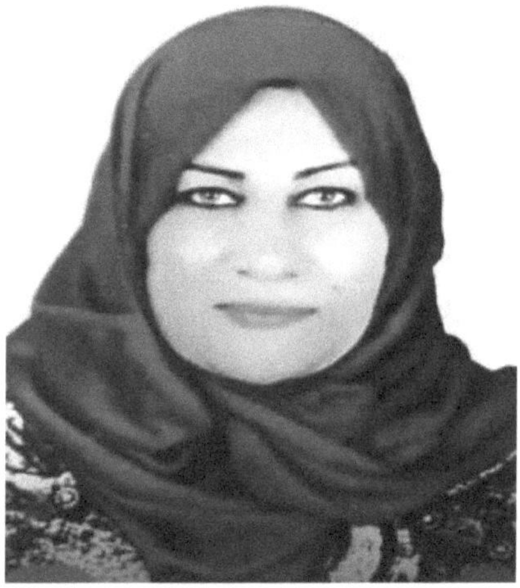

Dr. Hawraa Mahmood Murad

Department of biology, College of science, Al-Qasim Green University, Iraq

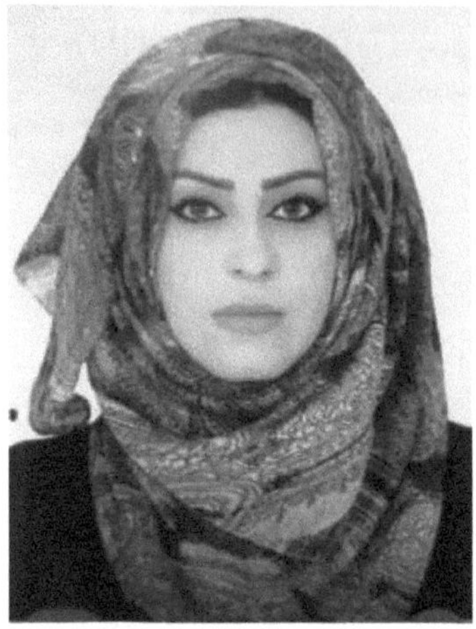

Dr. Rawaa Safaa Abbas AL_Azzawi

Department of biology, Collage of science, Al-Qasim Green University, Iraq

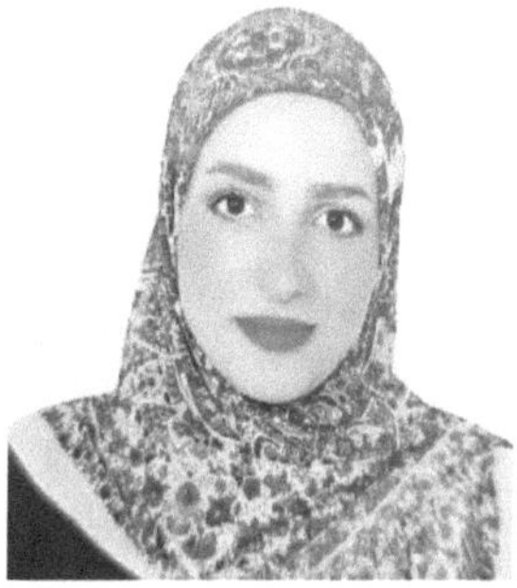

Dr. Mariam Kazim Jassab

Internal and Preventive Medicine College of Veterinary Medicine Al-Qasim Green University, Iraq

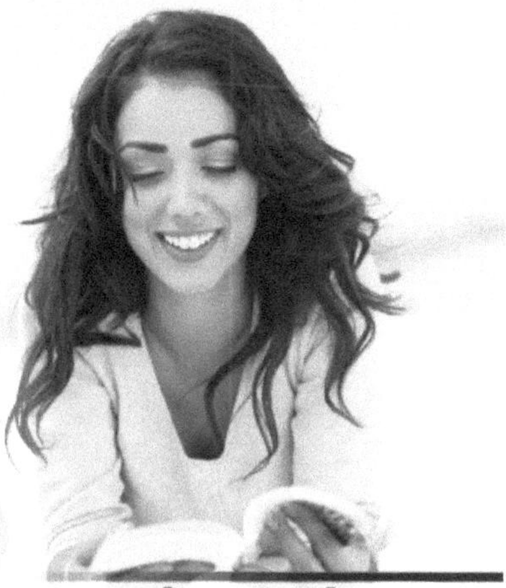

FSC
www.fsc.org
MIX
Papier | Fördert
gute Waldnutzung
FSC® C083411

Kolibri 360 GmbH
Ferdinand-Jühlke-Straße 7
99095 Erfurt, Deutschland
produktsicherheit@kolibri360.de

Druck:
CPI Druckdienstleistungen GmbH
im Auftrag der
Kolibri 360 GmbH
Ferdinand-Jühlke-Str. 7
99095 Erfurt